Preventive Dentistry

Preventive Dentistry

Leon M. Silverstone
B.CH.D, LDSRCS (ENG.), PH.D, DD.SC

Professor and Head, Division of Cariology, Dows Institute for Dental Research and Professor of Pedodontics, College of Dentistry, University of Iowa, USA

1978
UPDATE BOOKS
LONDON/FORT LEE

Available in the United Kingdom and Eire from
Update Books Ltd
33/34 Alfred Place
London WC1E 7DP
England

Available outside the United Kingdom from
Update Publishing International Inc.
2337 Lemoine Avenue
Fort Lee, New Jersey 07024
USA

First published 1978

British Library Cataloguing in Publication Data

Silverstone, Leon M
  Preventive dentistry
  1. Preventive dentistry
  I. Title
  617.6'01   RK60.7
  ISBN 0-906141-06-0

ISBN 0 906141 06 0

Printed in Great Britain by Cox & Wyman Ltd.
Fakenham, Norfolk

Contents

Preface

Dental disease accounts for more pain, suffering and loss of working hours than almost any other disease. And yet, since no one dies as a result of dental disease and since tooth loss is still regarded incorrectly as a normal consequence of ageing, there has been no major emphasis towards or demands for the preventive aspect of dentistry. By tradition, dentistry has been largely a reparative profession. However, reparative dentistry alone cannot bring about the control of dental disease which has now reached epidemic proportions in some countries. Over the past decade, the results of basic research, applied research and clinical trials from many parts of the world have shown that preventive dentistry can be highly successful.

This book deals with the prevention of dental caries and has been written for the dental practitioner, the dental student, the postgraduate worker and those engaged in dental research. Basic knowledge of the disease mechanisms, the tissues they affect and the scientific basis for each preventive technique described have been presented. Preventive dentistry requires a team approach; the dentist being the leader, with the other ancillary workers acting as important members of the team.

This book is also intended for hygienists and all other ancillary dental workers because, if prevention is to be accomplished successfully, it is essential that all members of the dental team are fully conversant with the philosophy and practice of preventive dentistry. In fact, all health delivery personnel, from the medical practitioner to the midwife, should have some knowledge of preventive dentistry and they too can benefit accordingly from this book.

In an attempt to keep this book to a reasonable size and not assume the proportions of a conventional textbook, the text has been kept to a minimum, illustrations used where possible and only key references given. Thus, this is not meant as an exhaustive work on the subject and therefore some areas may have been omitted or dealt with more superficially. Emphasis has been given to the practical and clinical aspects of caries prevention which the author feels to be of prime importance and for which there is a scientific basis.

Leon M. Silverstone

1. Dental Caries: The Problem

In recent years there has been a growing interest in preventive aspects of dentistry. Initially it is difficult for the dental practitioner to become preventive orientated. Perhaps the main reason is that if prevention is to be effective, the dentist himself must believe that prevention works. This is probably the most difficult concept for him to accept because throughout his undergraduate and other training the reparative aspects of dentistry were stressed, and the major part of his practice time is almost certainly spent on tooth repair. In addition, the high level of dental disease to which the practitioner is continually exposed, together with the relative absence of any formal training, knowledge or experience in preventive dentistry, will tend to impress upon him that the prevention of dental disease is more of an academic rather than a practical approach to the problem.

Therefore, the first essential step towards practising preventive dentistry is a change in basic philosophy. Prevention is not the purchasing of a topical fluoride kit. This may be one important item used in caries prevention, but it is secondary to the philosophy of preventive dentistry to be adopted by the dentist himself. Dental diseases can be prevented—prevention does work.

To practise competent preventive dentistry it is necessary to have some basic knowledge of the disease mechanisms and the tissues they affect. Only by understanding the essential points in the initiation and progress of the disease one is attempting to prevent can the best be derived out of preventive techniques. In addition, it is also possible to adopt a critical approach in the evaluation of laboratory and clinical tests of new preventive materials and techniques reported in the dental literature.

This does not imply that reparative procedures are to be forgotten. On the contrary, if the dental profession is to prevent or control dental disease, reparative treatment must be carried out alongside prevention. By looking at the dental problems of other countries which are fortunate in having a more favourable dentist–population ratio, such as in Scandinavia, it is obvious that reparative treatment alone cannot bring about the control of dental disease.

In this book the author will attempt to cover a number of aspects of caries prevention that can be adopted in general dental practice. In this chapter relevant factors in the basic disease process will be discussed and attention focused on the surface of the tooth. This will form an important part of the scientific basis for preventive dentistry.

Epidemiology of Dental Caries

Dental caries is a disease affecting almost the entire toothbearing population, and in the UK less than two per cent of the dentate population is free of the disease. There is a high level of caries in the deciduous dentition, represented by a range of four to five dmf teeth involved at five years of age. By 12 years of age, 25 per cent of the teeth of the population as a whole has become affected. Berman (1970) in a three-year study of schoolgirls between 11 and 15 years of age in the counties of Essex and Kent in England showed that by 15 years of age the majority had at least 10 DMF teeth. The adult dental health survey carried out in England and Wales (Gray et al. 1970) showed that only three adults in 1,000 had not suffered from dental caries at sometime in their lives. In addition, 38 per cent of the population over the age of 16 years had no teeth left at all. In the USA, by the age of 20 years, 15 teeth have been affected by dental caries and yet only eight have been restored. Of the seven remaining, two are carious and five are missing. Sheiham and Hobdell (1969) showed that the DMF index rose from 11, for 15- to 19-year-olds, to 25.8 for persons aged 60 to 65 years of age. However, as Jackson (1961) has indicated, the DMF index becomes less accurate as a measure of caries experience after 25 years of age, because periodontal disease then becomes a major factor in tooth loss. Epidemiological data thus provide evidence that the first two decades of life present a period of very high caries activity.

The Small Carious Lesion

Figure 1 shows a premolar tooth which was extracted for orthodontic purposes. Before extraction, the tooth was examined very carefully for caries. Clinical examination using a mirror and an explorer detected no lesion on either the occlusal or interstitial surfaces. There was no evidence of damage to unwaxed dental floss when passed between the contact points. Bite-wing radiographs were taken at normal, double and treble exposure times and examined on an illuminated viewer with a magnifying glass. No evidence of approximal caries was found, even on the radiographs taken with longer exposure times. The tooth was therefore diagnosed as being

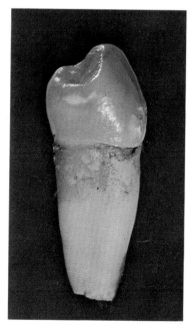

Figure 1. *A premolar tooth showing a 'white spot' carious lesion on the approximal surface.*

caries-free and extracted under local analgesia. However, on examining the extracted and dried tooth (Figure 1), a small white region can be seen on the approximal surface with no apparent difficulty. This is the 'white spot' lesion, which is the earliest macroscopic evidence of caries. The enamel surface overlying the lesion is intact and well mineralized and no difference between this surface and the adjacent sound enamel can be detected with an explorer. The reason for this is that in the small enamel lesion, demineralization occurs predominantly at a subsurface level. The surface overlying the lesion remains intact and well mineralized. This fascinating feature of the small enamel lesion can be shown in the laboratory by preparing thin, undecalcified, ground sections through the lesion.

Figure 2 shows a longitudinal ground section through the same lesion examined by transmitted light microscopy. The tooth section is not permanently fixed to the glass slide but is stored in water, and can be examined in any mounting medium. In Figure 2 the section is examined in quinoline, a medium similar to Canada balsam and having a refractive index identical to that of the enamel (1.62). The first important feature to be seen is the extent of the

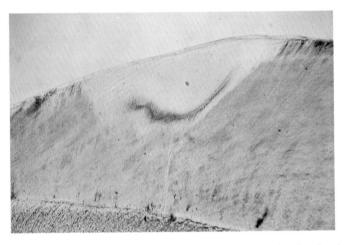

Figure 2. *Longitudinal ground section through the lesion shown in Figure 1. The section is examined in quinoline with transmitted light.*

lesion; it has penetrated approximately half-way through the enamel.

Figure 3 shows the identical field of view but this time examined with the polarizing microscope. The relevance of this technique will become apparent later on. Another simple technique which can be used to obtain relevant information from such a ground section is microradiography. A laboratory radiograph is taken of the tooth section on a glass plate covered with high resolution film. When developed, this microradiograph can then be examined with the light microscope. The radiographic technique employed differs from clinical radiography because soft x-rays are used (Cu Kα radiation).

Figure 4 is a microradiograph of the tooth section examined by low-power microscopy. The radiolucent demineralized area can be seen confined to the subsurface enamel, the enamel surface appearing intact and relatively well mineralized. Further studies showed that about 25 per cent of mineral had been lost from the subsurface region. The intact surface layer overlying the lesion had also been demineralized, but only to a level showing about one per cent of mineral loss.

Therefore, the most significant feature is that the carious lesion

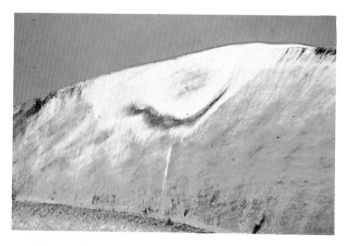

Figure 3. *Same field of view as in Figure 2 seen with the polarizing microscope.*

5

was not detected by clinical or radiographic means, although it had penetrated half-way through the enamel and about 25 per cent of tooth mineral had been removed by dissolution. This gives an idea of the size of the problem associated with the diagnosis of the small carious lesion. The clinician is only able to diagnose lesions that are already well advanced into the tooth. Our laboratory studies show that histologically the lesion must penetrate just into the dentine before evidence of a carious lesion is available on a routine bite-wing radiograph. At this stage, the lesion is observed on the radiograph as a small triangular region of radiolucency in the outer enamel.

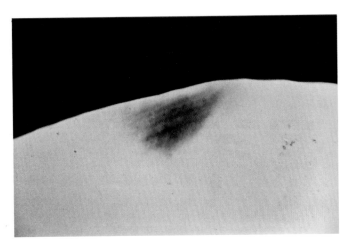

Figure 4. *Microradiograph of the same lesion showing the more heavily demineralized subsurface region. Note the well mineralized surface layer above the lesion.*

Figure 5 shows a similar 'white spot' lesion on the approximal surface of a deciduous molar. This lesion too was not detected by clinical or radiographic means. In the deciduous dentition the problem is even more acute. Instead of interstitial 'contact points' as in the permanent dentition, deciduous molars tend to have 'contact areas' because of their flattened approximal surfaces. Lesions are even more difficult to detect by clinical means than in the permanent dentition. In addition, enamel in deciduous teeth is about half the thickness of that in permanent teeth and the pulp chambers are relatively much larger. Thus, the carious process need travel a much shorter distance to reach the pulp in a deciduous molar relative to a permanent tooth. A number of studies have also shown that the rate of progress of a lesion is much faster through deciduous enamel compared with an equal distance in permanent enamel. It is possible, therefore, for caries to reach the pulp chamber in a deciduous tooth before there is clinical evidence of the presence of the lesion.

The enamel surface must therefore be regarded as the most important part of the tooth for the following reasons:

1. This is the only region that is available to the clinician for direct examination.

2. The carious process begins at the enamel surface.

3. The application of preventive materials must be made to the surface of the tooth.

Because of this, it is relevant to look a little more closely at the carious process with special reference to the enamel surface. This will constitute an important part of the scientific basis for caries prevention.

The Aetiology of Dental Caries

Dental plaque is now well recognized as playing a major role in the aetiology of dental caries and periodontal disease. In the mouth it is very difficult to obtain a clean enamel surface because the integuments of plaque penetrate some micrometres into the enamel surface. Soon after carrying out a thorough rubber-cup prophylaxis on accessible tooth surfaces, using pumice paste, a thin organic cuticle is rapidly deposited on the enamel. This is derived from saliva, containing essentially salivary mucopolysaccharides. This bacteria-free organic layer thickens (called a pellicle when about one micrometre thick) and it is into this matrix that oral bacteria become deposited. In addition to this build-up on clean smooth surfaces, there are numerous regions where the integrity of the enamel surface is deficient. Such regions can be identified readily when the enamel surface is examined by electron

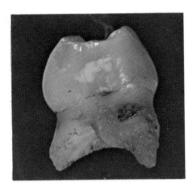

Figure 5. *A 'white spot' carious lesion on the approximal surface of a deciduous molar tooth.*

microscopy. It is almost impossible to remove colonies of bacteria from these sites (Figure 6). Thus, further build-up of plaque progresses rapidly from such 'wedge-defects' (Figure 7).

Although a great deal of research has been carried out, the precise aetiology of dental caries is still unresolved. There are three classical theories of caries aetiology. The acidogenic theory was proposed by Miller (1890) who stated that acids are produced at or near the tooth surface by bacterial fermentation of dietary carbohydrates. The acids are responsible for the dissolution of the apatite crystals which make up approximately 95 per cent of the bulk of the enamel. The proteolysis theory was proposed by Gottlieb (1944) who suggested that the initial attack on the enamel might be proteolytic rather than by acid. Human enamel contains less than one per cent of protein by weight, forming a delicate network coating the crystal surfaces. The theory proposes that proteolytic enzymes liberated by the oral bacteria could destroy the organic matrix of enamel. The proteolysis–chelation theory, originated by Schatz and Martin (1955), proposes that some of the products of bacterial action on enamel, dentine, food and salivary constituents may have the property of forming complexes or chelates with calcium. The theory suggests the possibility that demineralization of enamel could arise without acid formation since chelation occurs at neutral and alkaline pH values. All available evidence supports the acidogenic theory.

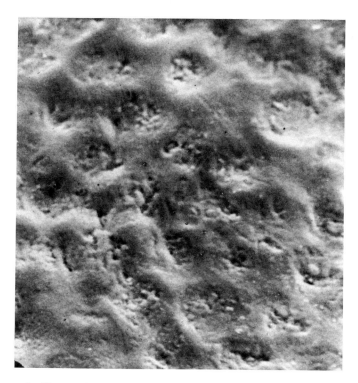

Figure 6. *Scanning electron micrograph of the enamel surface showing depressions which contain colonies of oral bacteria. Each depression corresponds with a prism thus being about 3—5 micrometres in width.*

The presence of bacteria in the mouth is essential to the production of caries, because it is bacterial enzymes which produce acid from carbohydrate. This was first proved by Orland and his colleagues (1954). Fitzgerald and Keyes (1960) established the infectious and transmissible nature of caries. Several strains isolated from human lesions have since been used to induce caries in monkeys maintained on a diet rich in sucrose and other carbohydrates but otherwise nutritionally adequate (Bowen 1969, pers. comm.). These organisms, and thus dental caries, are readily transferred from mother to offspring (Bowen 1968). The cariogenicity of the streptococci apparently lies in their ability to produce

9

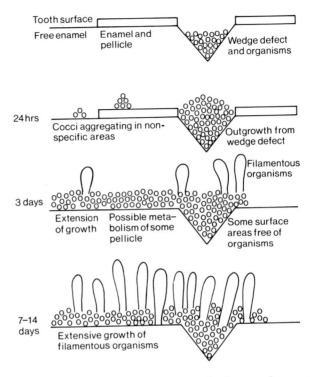

Figure 7. *Diagram showing stages of plaque formation.*

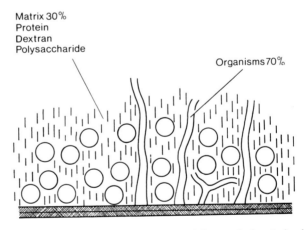

Figure 8. *Diagram showing composition of dental plaque.*

large amounts of extracellular polysaccharides from ingested sugars (Critchley et al. 1967). These extracellular polysaccharides (e.g. dextran) provide a sticky mass which enables plaque to adhere to the tooth surface (Figure 8). Acid subsequently produced in this plaque is prevented from diffusing away from the tooth by the plaque gel and at the same time prevented from being neutralized by salivary buffers. However, Bowen (1969) has shown that 24 hour old plaque has little capacity to lower the pH of a sugar solution. The capacity increases with age of the plaque, the maximum being reached after approximately three days.

The Special 'Surface Zone' Overlying the Small Carious Lesion

Although organic acids such as lactic acid are believed to be involved in caries formation, the use of these acids on enamel in the laboratory produces changes unlike those seen in caries.

Figure 9 shows the effect of exposing enamel to dilute lactic acid for several hours. The enamel surface has been grossly damaged by

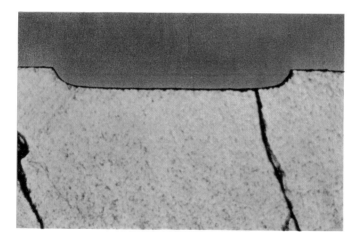

Figure 9. *Longitudinal ground section through a region of enamel that was exposed to dilute lactic acid, showing gross etching.*

11

etching, unlike the appearance of an intact surface seen in the small carious lesion. However, lactic acid can be used in the laboratory to produce lesions rather than just surface etching. This is achieved by

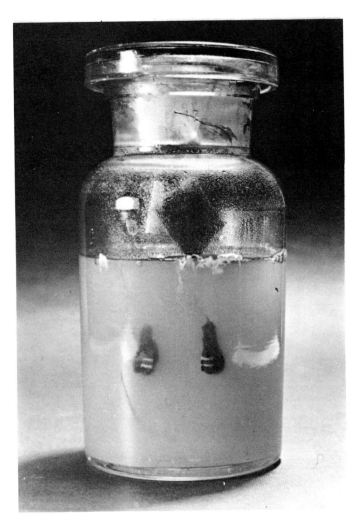

Figure 10. *Two teeth suspended in an acidified gel 'artificial caries' medium. The teeth are painted with coloured varnish except for window regions left exposed for experiment.*

adding other ions to the acid to slow down demineralization. If the acid is suspended in a gel, artificial lesions can be produced which appear indistinguishable from enamel caries when examined by light and electron microscopy (Silverstone 1967). Whereas the acid alone produces an etch within a matter of hours, months are required to produce a small 'white spot' lesion when the acid is used in a suitable gel matrix.

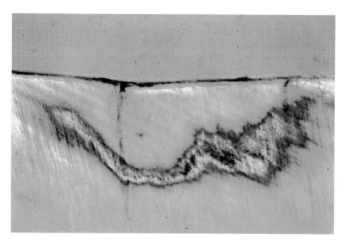

Figure 11. *Longitudinal ground section showing an artificial lesion produced in the acidified gel after five months' exposure. The lesion, examined in quinoline with polarized light, shows a dark zone at its advancing front and appears indistinguishable from enamel caries.*

Figure 10 shows two teeth suspended in an acidified gel, consisting of lactic acid and gelatin. The teeth have been painted with a coloured varnish to protect them, with the exception of small 'window' regions left unpainted for lesion formation. Figure 11 is a ground section through such an artificial lesion produced after five months' exposure. The lesion is examined in quinoline with the polarizing microscope and shows the characteristic histological features of enamel caries. If the same section is now examined in a different mounting medium, having a lower refractive index, a great deal of information can be obtained. Figure 12 is the same section examined in water. Under these conditions regions showing a yellow-brown colour (positive birefringence) have more than five per cent of mineral removed by dissolution. Although the subsurface region is heavily demineralized, the surface layer overlying the lesion is seen to retain the blue-green colour of normal enamel (negative birefringence). If the same histological 'trick' is repeated, a contour of the lesion can be built up showing levels of

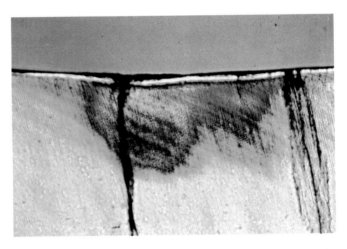

Figure 12. *Same section as in the previous figure showing the artificial lesion examined in water. The surface layer is relatively unaffected and shows the blue–green colour of sound enamel (negative birefringence).*

demineralization. Figure 13 once again shows the same section, but this time examined dry in air, the lowest possible refractive index. Under these conditions it requires a mineral loss of one per cent to change the blue–green colour to yellow–brown. The special 'surface zone' still shows the blue–green colour, indicating that it has only approximately one per cent mineral loss. Further studies show that the subsurface region has about 30 per cent of mineral removed.

Eventually, this relatively unaffected surface zone becomes

14

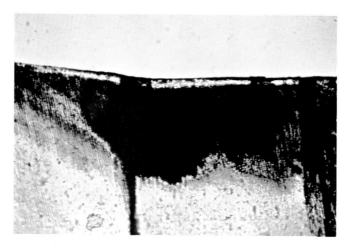

Figure 13. *Same section as in the previous two figures now examined dry in air. The surface zone still shows the blue–green colour of sound enamel indicating only about one per cent of mineral loss. The subsurface region has about 30 per cent of mineral loss.*

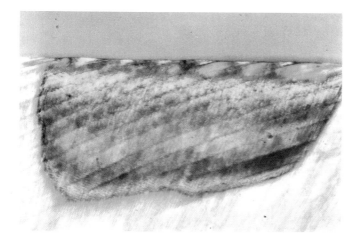

Figure 14. *A lesion showing the demineralization of the special surface zone. This is seen as yellow–brown streaks passing through the previously sound (blue–green) surface layer.*

15

demineralized; this is seen in Figure 14 as yellow–brown bands of demineralization passing through the surface layer. After this, the rate of progress of the lesion increases significantly (Silverstone 1968). The special surface layer is therefore a very important part of the lesion. It is because of its presence that small lesions are difficult to detect clinically. In addition, it controls to a large extent the rate of progress of the lesion. It has been shown in vitro (in the laboratory) that if the surface layer above a lesion can be further 'strengthened', the lesion may then become arrested or even reversed by remineralization (Silverstone 1972). This is of special significance in preventive dentistry because the application of preventive agents to the enamel surface can have a beneficial effect, not only on caries-free surfaces, but also on regions already carious.

Why is there a Surface Zone in the Small Carious Lesion?

Many workers have attributed the presence of a surface zone above the small lesion to the special properties of surface enamel.

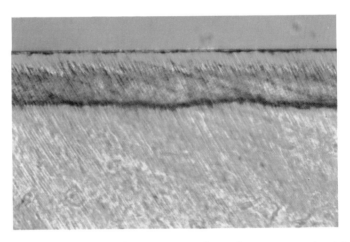

Figure 15. *An artificial lesion produced on enamel which had been artificially ground down before experiment. About 250 micrometres was cut away. However, there is still a well mineralized surface zone above the lesion.*

The surface has more fluoride than the subsurface enamel, it has less water, less carbonate, is more highly mineralized, and the enamel crystals are often larger and orientated differently from those below. This surface layer has special physical and chemical properties and is approximately 20 μm in depth. These factors without doubt make the enamel surface more resistant to acid attack than the subsurface region. However, these are not the only factors responsible. If the outer enamel surface, containing the special properties just mentioned, is cut away and an artificial lesion produced on the remaining surface, the lesion will still show a relatively unaffected surface zone (Silverstone 1968).

Figure 15 shows a lesion created on an enamel surface after cutting off 250 μm of enamel using a diamond wheel. The section is examined in water and yet the surface layer still shows a blue–green colour, the surface zone. Figure 16 is a micro-radiograph of another artificial lesion produced after 40 weeks in

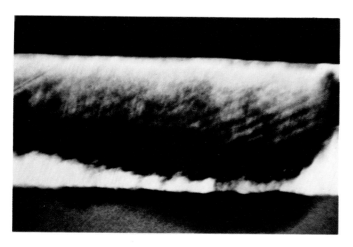

Figure 16. *This artificial lesion was produced after 40 weeks in the acidified gel medium. Before experiment, about 500 micrometres of the surface was removed. In spite of this, the surface still appears relatively unaffected while the subsurface region shows a high degree of mineral loss. The underlying dentine has also been demineralized.*

17

an acidified gel. Before the experiment $500\,\mu$m of the surface enamel was artificially abraded away (about half the thickness of enamel). However, the lesion still shows a well mineralized surface zone overlying the heavily demineralized subsurface region. The appearance of a surface zone is not therefore dependent upon the special properties of the enamel surface. It appears to be formed by 'remineralization' whereby dissolved ions from the subsurface region become deposited into the surface layer (Silverstone 1977).

This once again demonstrates the importance of the enamel surface in caries formation, and therefore in the prevention of the disease. The addition of fluoride ions to the surface above the lesion favours remineralization, and so helps maintain the integrity of the surface zone. This in turn will act as a 'brake' on the progress of the lesion. These factors must be appreciated by the preventive dentist in order to succeed in either preventing or arresting the carious lesion.

References

Berman, D. S., Ph.D. thesis, University of London, 1970.

Bowen, W. H., In *Advances in Oral Biology*, Vol. 3 (Ed. P. Staple) Academic Press, London, 1968.

Bowen, W. H., *Br. Dent. J.*, 1969, **126**, 159.

Critchley, P. et al., *Caries Res.*, 1967, **1**, 112.

Fitzgerald, R. J. and Keyes, P. H., *J. Am. Dent. Assoc.*, 1960, **61**, 9.

Gottlieb, B., *J. Dent. Res.*, 1944, **23**, 379.

Gray, P. G., Todd, J. E., Slack, G. L. and Bulman, J. S., *Adult Dental Health in England and Wales in 1968*, HMSO, London, 1970.

Jackson, D., *Arch. Oral Biol.*, 1961, **6**, 80.

Miller, W. D., *The Micro-organisms of the Human Mouth*, White Dental Manufacturing Co., Philadelphia, 1890.

Orland, F. J. et al., *J. Dent. Res.*, 1954, **33**, 147.

Schatz, A. and Martin, J. J., *N.Y. State Dent. J.*, 1955, **21**, 367.

Shieham, A. and Hobdell, M. H., *Brit. Dent. J.*, 1969, **126**, 401.

Silverstone, L. M., Ph.D. thesis, University of Bristol, 1967.

Silverstone, L. M., *Brit. Dent. J.*, 1968, **125**, 145.

Silverstone, L. M., *Proc. Roy. Soc. Med.*, 1972, **65**, 906.

Silverstone, L. M., *Caries Res.*, 1977, **11** (Suppl 1), 59.

2. Systemic Fluoride

Trendley Dean and his co-workers (1942) carried out extensive epidemiological studies on children between 12 and 14 years of age in 20 towns in the USA relating caries experience and the fluoride content of the drinking water. They showed that if the domestic water supply contained about 1 ppm of fluoride, a nearly maximal reduction in the mean caries rate was observed, and yet hypoplasia of enamel was no higher than in areas with little or no fluoride in the water.

A comparison of the mean caries experience in children living in areas where the water contained 1 ppm of fluoride with others having little or no fluoride showed a reduction of well over 50 per cent. The conclusive demonstration of these beneficial effects from a number of studies led to the proposal that the fluoride content of water supplies deficient in this element should be adjusted to a level giving a maximal reduction in caries without producing mottling. In temperate climates this is approximately 1 ppm of fluoride. Such a public health measure presents no technical difficulties and is inexpensive to carry out.

Since 1945 when fluoride was first added to a domestic water supply to test its effect on caries incidence, many experimental studies have been initiated. Reports on the effects of artificial fluoridation of water are thus available for periods of up to 25 years, and confirm that the benefits are similar to those produced by water naturally fluoridated at the same concentration. The major fluoridation studies which have been carried out in various parts of the world have been reviewed recently (Murray 1976).

Throughout the world about 130 million people in 33 countries receive the benefits of fluoridated drinking water. This shows the importance that many countries place on the need for the prevention of dental caries, and on the effectiveness of fluoride as a public health measure. The efficacy and safety of fluoride has been proved beyond doubt. In the UK, however, only about 3 million people receive fluoridated water (six per cent of the population). In contrast, approximately 105 million people in the USA receive water supplies that are fluoridated either naturally or artificially (59 per cent of the population). However, approximately 40 million people in the USA live in rural areas not receiving community water supplies and therefore cannot benefit from fluoridation.

The Effects on the Teeth of Water Fluoridation

Originally it was believed that the only teeth to benefit were those calcifying and maturing during the period of drinking fluoridated water. It is now known that fluoride lowers the subsequent

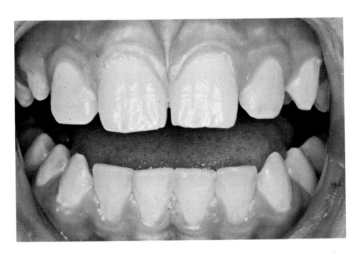

Figure 17. *A caries-free mouth in a child, 12 years of age living in a region where the water contains fluoride at a level of 1 ppm. Note the excellent appearance of the hard and shiny enamel with no evidence of opaque spots or intrinsic stains.*

experience of smooth surface caries even of those teeth which had been erupted for a few years before the institution of fluoridation.

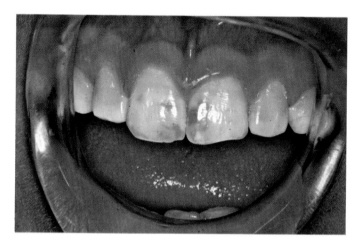

Figure 18. *A case of enamel fluorosis (mottling) in an area containing 3 to 4 ppm fluoride in the domestic water.*

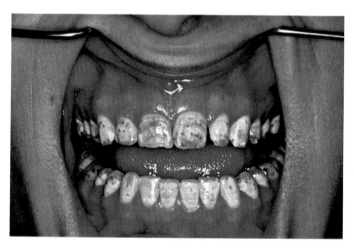

Figure 19. *This severe case of enamel fluorosis occurred in India in a region containing about 6 ppm fluoride in the drinking water. Note the enamel hypoplasia in addition to staining.*

It is still widely believed that the administration of fluorides prenatally is of significant value. However, there is little evidence to support this claim, even in the deciduous dentition. Recent work has shown that there is little or no passage of fluoride through the

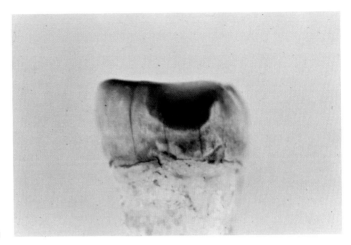

a

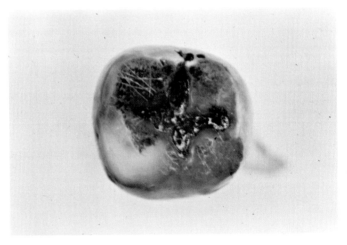

b

Figure 20. *(a) and (b) A molar tooth from a Turkish patient reared in an area containing 5 ppm fluoride in the water. Buccal and occlusal views of the tooth show extensive staining. The tooth is caries-free and was lost from this elderly patient because of periodontal disease.*

placenta in the monkey (Bowen 1976, pers. comm.). Thus, the evidence available does not give clear support to the use of fluoride as a prenatal supplement for caries prevention in children. In general, the greatest benefits of natural and artificial fluoridation are observed in the incidence of caries on smooth surfaces.

Economic Aspects of Water Fluoridation

The cost of adjusting the fluoride concentration of water supplies is inexpensive. Fluoridation costs between seven and ten pence (15 to 20 cents) per resident per year and even if prorated only amongst children, the cost is only about 25p (50 cents) per child annually.

Mottling of Teeth

Enamel fluorosis (mottling) of the permanent teeth results from the ingestion of water containing more than 2 ppm of fluoride in the drinking water during the first 10 years of life. Once enamel formation has been completed, mottling cannot occur. The degree of mottling varies from small opaque white spots covered by an intact, hard and shiny surface, to gross dark-brown lesions with a pitted surface. The severity is directly related to the fluoride level of the domestic water. Mottling is insignificant below 2 ppm of fluoride (Figure 17). In fact, the community index of hypoplastic defects in enamel is at its minimum when the fluoride level of the water is at 1 ppm (Forrest and James 1965), the implication being that fluoride at this level produces a more perfect enamel structure. Staining does not occur until a concentration of 3 to 4 ppm of fluoride is reached (Figure 18), with gross lesions appearing at 5 to 7 ppm of fluoride (Figures 19 and 20).

Fluoridation of Salt and Milk

Domestic salt is used in all households and has therefore been advocated as an alternative vehicle for fluoride. It has already been employed for ensuring an adequate intake of iodine in areas deficient in this element. Data on the variation in the consumption of domestic salt is not so thoroughly documented as that of water. As a result it has not so far been practical to ensure a satisfactory mean dose for a population without incurring the possibility of an overdose for the few. In Switzerland, fluoridated salt is available in many cantons, but the level of fluoride is usually reduced to provide a mean daily dose of about one-third of that received from water fluoridated at the 1 ppm level. After five years of salt fluoridation, caries incidence in children between seven and 12 years of age was reduced significantly, but the reduction was only about half of that to be expected after water fluoridation. More precise data on the variation in salt intake within communities may enable the level of fluoride in salt to be increased without the possibility of toxic hazard for the few. In the present state of knowledge, the effects of fluoridated salt on dental caries are unlikely to equal those from water fluoridation. However, a significant proportion of the world's population does not have access to a piped water supply. Therefore, an alternative vehicle for fluoride must be available for such regions. Detailed studies on the use of fluoridated salt have also been carried out in Colombia, South America, and are in progress in Hungary.

A small number of investigations have been undertaken to assess the effectiveness of fluoridated milk. These studies have not been as extensive as those with domestic salt but appear to indicate benefits similar to those arising from the fluoridation of salt. Because of the relatively large number of distribution centres for milk in most countries, in practice this method might be more expensive and less easy to implement than fluoridation of either salt or water. However, an ingenious milk fluoridation plant has been designed in the UK (Borrow 1971) which can supply, in a simple three-stage process, milk fluoridated to any specific level. Research being carried out now may produce significant findings.

Fluoride Tablets

Fluoride tablets chewed or sucked as a preventive measure would be expected to combine some of the benefits arising locally, because of topical application on erupted teeth, with systemic effects because of the ingestion of fluoride and its effects on unerupted teeth. If the regimen is conscientiously adhered to, it will provide a consistent dose of fluoride. However, it is not a public health measure and only a relatively small number of parents among the 'regular attenders' are motivated enough to use it today. In addition, it has two inherent disadvantages. First, it calls for intelligent co-operation from the parents, and second, the tablets must be kept in a safe place out of reach of children who might be tempted to ingest a large number. However, today fluoride tablets are the only practical alternative to the consumption of fluoridated water. Because the systemic use of fluoride is a highly significant factor in caries prevention, the ingestion of an optimum level of fluoride during tooth development must form the basis for any successful caries preventive regimen. A number of parents ask their medical practitioner for advice on the use of fluoride tablets. They are often told that such a procedure is not really necessary. Such advice must come from the dental practitioner, and not just when the parent requests it. Therefore, it is essential that the dental practitioner knows all the relevant factors relating to the use of fluoride tablets. In this way he can better motivate his patients to use them for their children and answer the many queries that he may receive from patients and professional colleagues. If he has not mentioned the use of fluoride tablets before the parents' request for information, and if he is unable to supply logical answers, then he can hardly instil confidence in this important preventive measure.

Recent information from several sources suggests that previous recommendations for fluoride supplementation of infants and small children may lead to greater intakes of fluoride than are desirable (Aasenden and Peebles 1974; Fanning et al. 1975; Fomon and Wei 1976; Forrester and Schulz 1974; Infante 1975; Wiatrowski et al. 1975).

Previous Recommendations

Recent information suggests that previous recommendations for fluoride supplementation may be higher than desirable and be responsible for the appearance of mild enamel fluorosis. The International Workshop on Fluoride and Dental Caries Reduction

(Forrester and Schulz 1974) recommended that fluoride supplementation should begin as soon after birth as possible and continue through the teenage years.

The Council on Dental Therapeutics of the American Dental Association (1973) recommends that no fluoride supplementation should be given if the fluoride level in the water supply exceeds 0.7 ppm. In fluoride deficient areas, where the local water supply contains less than 0.2 ppm fluoride, the following is recommended. For infants, one 2.2 mg tablet of sodium fluoride (1 mg fluoride ion) should be dissolved in one quart of drinking water to provide fluoridated water which can be used for drinking and the preparation of infant foods. For children between two and three years of age, one 2.2 mg tablet of sodium fluoride may be given every other day, or half a tablet given daily.

The Committee on Nutrition of the American Academy of Pediatrics (1972) recommends 0.5 mg fluoride ion per day for children up to age three years and 1.0 mg daily after this age for residents of fluoride deficient communities.

Aasenden and Peebles (1974) reported that 67 per cent of children on fluoride supplements conforming to the above levels have mild to very mild fluorosis of permanent teeth. Fourteen per cent of these children were in the moderate category but no discolouration or pitting of the enamel was seen. The authors recommended that consideration·be given to reducing the dosage prior to age three years and increasing the dosage after five to six years of age when formation of tooth crowns of anterior teeth is almost complete.

Hotz (1974) reported similar observations of mild enamel fluorosis in Switzerland when children received 0.5 mg fluoride ion from birth to four years of age and 1.0 mg thereafter. As a result the fluoride supplementation regimen has been modified in Switzerland.

New Recommendations

Fomon and Wei (1976) have suggested that no supplementation be used during the first six months of life, and that fluoride supplementation be introduced thereafter in increments of 0.25 mg

(Table 1). The author recommends this new supplementation schedule.

Table 1. Recommended fluoride supplementation.

Fluoride concentration of water supply (ppm)	Age 0–6 months	Age 6–18 months	Age 18–36 months	Age 3–6 years	Age >6 years
<0.2	0	0.25	0.5	0.75	1.0
0.2–0.4	0	0	0.25	0.50	0.75
0.4–0.6	0	0	0	0.25	0.50
0.6–0.8	0	0	0	0	0.25
>0.8	0	0	0	0	0

(Data from Fomon and Wei 1976.)

Birth to Six Months of Age

Recent data suggest that many infants may receive more dietary fluoride than was previously thought (Wiatrowski et al. 1975). In addition, the fluoride content of commercially prepared concentrated liquid formulae may vary widely even amongst products produced by the same manufacturer. Whether a single daily dose of the appropriate level of fluoride beginning at birth confers a greater protection against dental caries than does an appropriate dose commencing at six months of life is unknown. Therefore, in view of this uncertainty and the difficulties in formulating an appropriate daily dose of fluoride for infants from birth to six months of age, it is suggested that fluoride supplementation be delayed until age six months (Fomon and Wei 1976).

Six Months to Eighteen Months of Age

Since infants probably receive greater intakes of fluoride from foods than was previously envisaged (Wiatrowski et al. 1975), the fluoride dosage of 0.5 mg daily previously recommended (Wei 1974) may be too high. Aasenden and Peebles (1974) have shown that children living in a community with a low fluoride concentration in the drinking water and who received a supplement of 0.5 mg fluoride daily from birth to three years and 1 mg thereafter

27

Preventive Dentistry

showed a significant caries reduction (80 per cent) compared with the controls. However, 67 per cent of the children were classified as having fluorosis of the very mild or mild type. Other investigators have also observed mild enamel fluorosis following this recommended dosage (Wei et al. 1977; see Chapter 10). Therefore, Fomon and Wei (1976) and Wei et al. (1977) have recommended a maximal daily dose of 0.25 mg of fluoride for children between 6 and 18 months of age (Table 1).

From Eighteen Months to Three Years of Age

Where the local water supply is deficient with respect to fluoride, having less than 0.2 ppm fluoride, a daily supplementation of 0.5 mg fluoride ion should be given. If the local water supply contains 0.2 to 0.4 ppm fluoride, the daily fluoride tablet should contain only 0.25 mg fluoride ion. If the local water supply contains more than 0.5 ppm fluoride, no additional fluoride should be given.

From Three to Six Years of Age

Where the local water supply contains less than 0.2 ppm fluoride, a daily supplementation of 0.75 mg fluoride ion should be given. If the local water supply contains 0.2 to 0.4 ppm fluoride, then the daily dosage should be reduced to 0.5 mg fluoride ion. No fluoride tablets should be given if the water supply contains 0.5 or more ppm fluoride.

From Six Years of Age

The full daily supplementation of 1.0 mg fluoride ion should be given if the fluoride concentration of the local drinking water is less than 0.2 ppm. Where the water supply contains 0.2 to 0.4 ppm fluoride, the daily dosage should be reduced to 0.75 mg fluoride ion. This should be further reduced to 0.5 mg fluoride ion daily if the local water supply contains 0.4 to 0.6 ppm fluoride. With a fluoride concentration of 0.6 to 0.8 ppm fluoride, the daily supplementation should be 0.25 mg fluoride ion. No supplementation should be given if the local water contains more than 0.8 ppm fluoride.

Fluoride Preparations and Methods of Application

Fluoride Tablets

Tablets containing sodium fluoride are available from many commercial sources and studies have shown that salivary fluoride concentrations approaching 200 ppm are obtained intraorally from chewing 2.2 mg sodium fluoride tablets (Parkins 1971; 1972).

In the USA, fluoride dosages have also been combined with the recommended daily dose of multivitamins. The products presently available contain 1.0 mg and 0.5 mg fluoride ion. Fluoride–vitamin tablets have been shown to have similar effects on dental caries to tablets containing fluoride alone (Hennon et al. 1972). As yet, 0.25 mg fluoride tablets which contain the recommended daily vitamin dosage are not marketed.

Ideally a fluoride tablet should be sucked in order to increase the topical fluoride effect. Stephen and Campbell (1978) demonstrated the topical fluoride effect of sucking a fluoride tablet on each school day, which produced a dramatic reduction in caries over a three-year period. Tablets that contain 0.25 mg fluoride ion should be available to comply with the new recommendations for fluoride supplementation (Table 1).

Fluoride Liquids or Drops

Liquid fluoride preparations are available which permit dispensing of controlled amounts of fluoride by a dropper. Usually 0.1 mg of fluoride per drop is dispensed. Drops should be placed on the tongue or inside the cheek where they are not swallowed directly or aspirated.

Fluoride Supplementation Commenced after Two Years of Age

At one time it was believed that significant benefits could only be achieved by receiving fluoride early on during the period of formation and calcification of the enamel matrix. However, studies after 10 years of water fluoridation have invalidated this earlier hypothesis (Marthaler 1967). If a child begins a systemic fluoride regimen after two years of age, or even later, significant benefit can still be achieved, especially on approximal tooth surfaces. It is only with respect to pit and fissure caries that systemic fluoride must begin soon after birth to have a beneficial effect. Even then, the preventive effect for occlusal caries is still much less than for other tooth surfaces (Backer Dirks 1963). It appears that there is a significant uptake of fluoride by the enamel surface within a period of about 12 months before eruption of a tooth. Of clinical relevance this means therefore that a child of four to five years of age can still begin a fluoride tablet regimen and obtain a beneficial effect, even with respect to the first permanent molars. In addition, the significant topical fluoride effect of sucking fluoride tablets has been demonstrated by Stephen and Campbell (1978).

Dangers

Parents should be warned that if several days or weeks go by without the child receiving fluoride tablets, they should not try to make up the deficiency by increasing the dose. This problem might arise, for example, if the parents forgot to take their fluoride tablets with them on holiday. They should be told that on restarting the regimen, the normal dose only should be given. Even though this is common sense, it should be stressed to every parent.

Fluoride tablets, like all other tablets and medicines, must be kept in a safe place and out of reach of children. If not, there is the danger of the child swallowing a number of tablets. If the parents of such a child contact their dental practitioner, he should first try to find out from the parents the approximate number of tablets taken. If it is just a few, then the child should be encouraged to drink a large volume of milk, the calcium ions thus helping to 'mop up' fluoride ions. Alternatively, 1 to 2 g calcium chloride or lactate, dissolved in water, may be given orally followed by an emetic. If the parents are not certain of the number, or if many have been taken, it is advisable to refer the child to hospital where a stomach wash will almost certainly be carried out.

References

Aasenden, R. and Peebles, T. C., *Arch. Oral Biol.*, 1974, **19**, 321.

American Dental Association, Prescribing fluoride supplements, in *Accepted Dental Therapeutics* (36 ed.), pp. 291–293, Chicago, 1973.

Backer Dirks, O., *Br. Dent. J.*, 1963, **114**, 211.

Borrow, E. W., *Water and Water Engineering*, 1971.

Committee on Nutrition, *Am. Acad. Pediatrics*, 1972, **49**, 456.

Dean, H. T., Arnold, F. A. and Elvove, E., *Publ. Hlth. Rep.* (Wash.), 1942, **57**, 1155.

Fanning, E. A., Cellier, K. M., Leadbeater, M. M. and Somerville, C. M., *Aust. Dent. J.* 1975, **20**, 7.

Fomon, S. J. and Wei, S. H. Y., in *Nutritional Disorders of Children* S. J. Fomon (Ed.), pp. 82–95, DHEW Pub. No. (HSA) 76–5612, 1976.

Forrest, J. R. and James, P. M. C., *Advances in Fluorine Research and Dental Caries Prevention* J. L. Hardwick, H. R. Held and K. G. Konig (Eds), Pergamon Press, Oxford, **3**, 233.

Forrester, D. J. and Schulz, E. M. jr. (Eds), *International Workshop on Fluorides and Dental Caries Reductions*, pp. 104–106, University of Maryland, Baltimore, 1974.

Hennon, D. K., Stookey, G. K. and Beiswanger, B. B., *Proc. IADR 54th Gen. Meeting, Miami 1972*, Abstr. No. 90, American Dental Association, Chicago..

Hotz, P., in *International Workshop on Fluorides and Dental Caries Reductions*, University of Maryland, Baltimore, 1974.

Infante, P. F., *Am. J. Dis. Child.*, 1975, **129**, 835.

Marthaler, T., *Int. Dent. J.*, 1967, **17**, 606.

Murray, J., *Fluorides in Caries Prevention*, J. J. Murray (Ed.), Dent. Pract. Handbook No. 20, John Wright, Bristol, 1976.

Parkins, F. M., *J. Dent. Res.*, 1971, **50**, 515.

Parkins, F. M., *J. Dent. Res.*, 1972, **51**, 1346.

Stephen, K. W. and Campbell, D., *Br. Dent. J.*, 1978, **144**, 202.

Wei, S. H. Y., in *Infant Nutrition*, S. J. Fomon (Ed.), pp. 338–358, W. B. Saunders, Philadelphia, 1974.

Wei, S. H. Y., Wefel, J. S. and Parkins, F. M., *J. Prev. Dent.*, 1977, **4**, 28.

Wiatrowski, E., Kramer, L., Osis, D. and Spencer, H., *Pediatrics*, 1975, **55**, 517.

3. Plaque Control

Research has indicated that dental caries does not develop in experimental animals fed their entire diet by stomach tube. However, Bowen (1969a) has shown that plaque still forms on tooth surfaces of monkeys in spite of receiving their diet in this manner. Bowen (1969a) further showed that the capacity of plaque to produce acid was influenced by the experimental regimen. When a normal cariogenic diet was fed by stomach tube for two weeks, almost no acid was formed in the plaque. Plaque formed in the presence of glucose had a much less acidogenic capacity than that formed from sucrose. Plaque formed three months after the animals had been returned to their normal diet had approximately the same acidogenic potential as that formed before the experiment.

Periodontal disease is the major cause of tooth loss after 35 years of age. In common with dental caries, periodontal disease is widespread. In one study 99 per cent of secondary schoolchildren were found to have some form of the disease and, by 17 years of age, 36 per cent had one or more true periodontal pocket (Sheiham 1969). From 35 to 39 years of age, 46 per cent of adults in the UK exhibit the terminal stages of periodontal disease and are about to lose teeth because of the disease. In those between 55 and 59 years of age, the percentage has increased to 95 per cent (Sheiham 1971). It has been shown (Löe et al. 1965) that clinical gingival inflammation can be eliminated by thorough toothbrushing. In addition, most periodontal disease can be controlled or prevented by oral hygiene practice aimed at the removal of plaque (Greene and Vermillion 1971).

Plaque Control

It is now well accepted that dental plaque is a major aetiological factor in the two main dental diseases—caries and periodontal disease. Plaque consists essentially of microcolonies of bacteria held in a gel-like matrix. The matrix is derived from the bacteria themselves, from saliva and, in areas adjacent to gingival tissue, from gingival fluid and inflammatory exudate. The mechanism of plaque formation has been mentioned in Chapter 1. Shortly after a polished tooth surface is exposed to saliva, a structureless organic pellicle forms. The first micro-organisms start to colonize it and a thin layer of bacterial plaque is formed within hours. After 24 hours without tooth cleansing, a clinically observable soft deposit is seen at the tooth–gingival margin interface. Plaque formation at the cervical margins is relatively independent of the passage of food orally. Hence, the concept of 'self-cleansing' on an ordinary diet does not exist in man. Tube-feeding is associated with as much plaque formation as chewing and swallowing. Excessive chewing of fibrous foods between meals cannot prevent the formation of plaque. Even if the bacteria which cause caries and periodontal disease are present in the mouth, they cannot initiate either disease process until they are able to attach themselves to the teeth in the

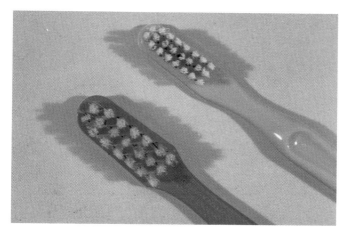

Figure 21. *Examples of suitable toothbrushes. The small brush is suitable for child or adult use.*

form of dental plaque. Thus, because plaque is such a significant factor in dental disease, its efficient removal must form a very important part of preventive dentistry.

Plaque control can be considered under the following headings:

1. Natural cleansing of the teeth.
2. Prophylaxis in the dental office.
3. Toothbrushing.
4. Dental flossing.
5. Oral rinsing.
6. Other devices.
7. Chemical control.
8. Diet.

Natural Cleansing of the Teeth

During mastication the interproximal and cervical areas of the tooth surface, the gingival margin and most of the attached gingiva are not cleaned effectively. Regular chewing of coarse foods has little effect on the accumulation of plaque in these sites. In addi-

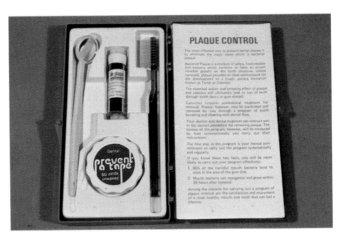

Figure 22. *A 'plaque control kit' containing toothbrush, disclosing agent, floss and mouth mirror.*

tion, neither the chewing of fibrous vegetables between meals nor the action of the tongue will prevent plaque from forming. In most developed countries natural cleansing of the teeth contributes little to oral hygiene and, consequently, if plaque is to be controlled, it must be removed actively. Today the physical removal of plaque is the only effective method, although research on chemical plaque control is in progress.

Prophylaxis in the Dental Office

The rubber-cup prophylaxis is an important factor in the introduction of dental procedures to children. From then on, a rubber-cup prophylaxis forms an integral part of oral hygiene instruction because it can demonstrate the effective removal of disclosed plaque from tooth surfaces. It also forms the initial stage in topical fluoride therapy and will be discussed in more detail in that context. However, because the professional prophylaxis is carried out infrequently, it is of relatively little value in the control of dental caries, although it may be of greater significance in the prevention of periodontal disease.

Toothbrushing

Human and animal experiments provide convincing evidence that accumulation of oral bacteria causes most common forms of periodontal disease. Löe et al. (1965) showed that complete cessation of oral hygiene results in gingivitis within two to three weeks. When oral hygiene procedures were then put into effect the gingivitis resolved. In clinical trials the relationship between caries and toothbrushing is less convincing than for periodontal disease. This may be because toothbrushing carried out in test groups is relatively inefficient, with the result that there is little difference compared with control groups not using brushing techniques. However, once a fluoride-containing dentifrice is used by a test group, small but significant caries reductions are shown.

First, the patient must be made aware of the nature of dental plaque, its formation, and significance in dental disease. Photographs or other types of visual aids can be used to advantage.

Toothbrushing techniques can then be demonstrated on models using suitable brushes (Figure 21). By repeating the various toothbrushing techniques on models, the patient can be familiarized with essential methods and made aware of the problems of cleaning interproximal regions and gingival margins. Oral hygiene instruction is then taken a stage further by application of the techniques to the patient's mouth.

It is essential to use a disclosing technique with dyes such as basic fuchsin or erythrosin, contained in either a disclosing tablet, capsule, wafer or fluid, many of which are now available (Figures 22, 23 and 24). When chewed and swished between the teeth for about 30 seconds, the dye is released and stains plaque a red colour (Figure 25). The dye does not stain clean tooth surfaces but will stain the tongue and lips for up to two hours. Staining of the lips can be prevented by coating them with vaseline. Plaque on soft tissues will also be stained. Food-colouring dyes may also be used in the same way. Recently, a disclosing fluid has been introduced which stains plaque differentially ('dis-plaque', Pacemaker Corporation). Thicker, old plaque stains blue which contrasts well

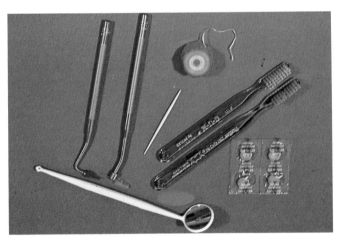

Figure 23. *Contents of another commercially available 'plaque control kit'. This one contains two brushes, disclosing tablets, floss, a mouth mirror and three types of interdental stimulators.*

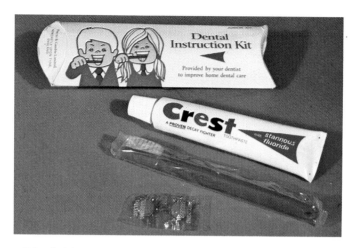

Figure 24. *A 'dental instruction kit' consisting of toothbrush, a fluoride-containing dentifrice and disclosing tablets.*

with teeth and soft tissues while thin, new plaque is stained red (Figure 26). This agent also fades much faster from soft tissues than conventional disclosing agents.

Efforts to develop staining methods which avoid observable red stains on the lips, tongue and gingiva have led to the introduction of fluorescent agents (Brilliant 1967; Hefferren et al. 1971). A system using this technique is available, known as 'Plak-Lite' (Int. Pharmaceutical Corp., Warrington, Pa. 18976, USA), Plak-Lite (Figure 27) consists of a fluorescent disclosing agent and a light source to make the agent visible. The solution has a light absorbency which lies within the frequencies of 200 to 540 nm. Plak-Lite transmits blue light in the frequency range 420–560 nm. The front of the apparatus consists of a mirror in which the patient examines his mouth for the detection of fluorescent plaque. Lang et al. (1972), showed that Plak-Lite revealed plaque on the teeth, tongue and gingiva. Clean teeth, plaque-free gingiva and oral mucosa did not fluoresce. The fluorescence, which was detected only with the special blue light source, lasted for about 20 minutes and disappeared within two hours. This was considered more

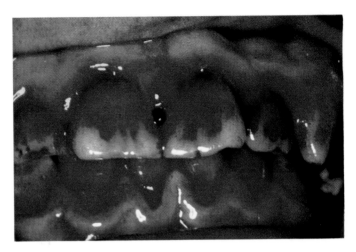

Figure 25. *Heavy and extensive deposits of dental plaque revealed after use of a disclosing agent. The erythrosin dye has stained almost all tooth surfaces including the gingival margins.*

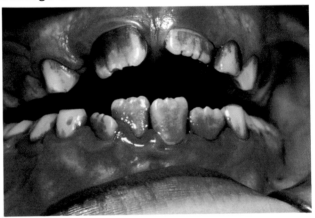

Figure 26. *Dis-plaque (Pacemaker Corp., Portland, Oregon) is a two-colour dental disclosing system. It stains differentially thick, older plaque in blue tones and thin, newer plaque red. Therefore, areas stained red are deposits built up within 24 hours of disclosing. This agent also fades faster from soft tissues than conventional disclosing agents.*

convenient for the patient than conventional disclosing agents. The Plak-Lite solution has a pleasant taste and is readily accepted by patients.

After using a disclosing technique the patient should clean his teeth over a basin, either in front of a mirror or using a hand mirror. After cleaning the patient should rinse out well and then dentist (or hygienist) and patient should carefully inspect the tooth surfaces. With the patient examining his mouth with the aid of a hand mirror, the instructor can point out areas which are still stained, and therefore retaining plaque. The patient should then brush his teeth again in an attempt to remove further stained areas, using a plastic dental mirror to inspect palatal and lingual surfaces.

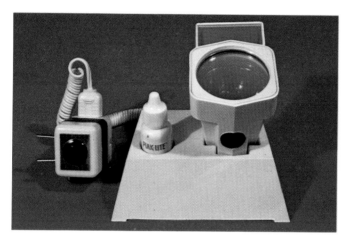

Figure 27. *The Plak-Lite kit.*

Motivating the Patient (and Parents)

One of the biggest drawbacks in effective toothbrushing is that it demands a high degree of patient co-operation. On average adults rarely brush their teeth for more than 30 seconds, and surfaces other than buccal and labial are often untouched. It has been shown that most children under five years of age brush for less than 20 seconds, and the only brushing zones are labial surfaces and the occlusal surfaces of lower molars (Kimmelmann and Tassman 1960).

Toothbrushing instruction by the dentist or his hygienist must appear enthusiastic to the adult or to the child and his parents, to motivate them to use the toothbrush frequently and correctly. Satisfactory results are not obtained by giving instruction sheets and pamphlets. Without trained inspection and supervision oral hygiene instruction fails. In the case of children success can only be achieved by direct supervision and participation by the parent.

The patient should use disclosing techniques at home and thus carry out his own assessment of oral hygiene levels. Dental-type plastic mouth mirrors are available in several 'plaque control kits' (Figures 22 and 23) which enable the patient to check on palatal and lingual surfaces. In addition to plastic dental mirrors, control kits contain items such as disclosing tablets, toothbrushes, unwaxed dental floss, interdental stimulators and wood sticks.

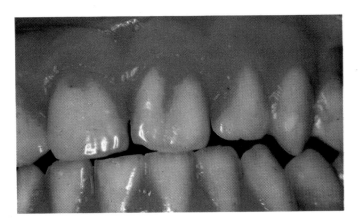

Figure 28. *In this case, the patient used a disclosing agent after carrying out careful toothbrushing. Many areas still show the retention of plaque, especially at the gingival margins. The use of disclosing agents after brushing, in this manner, is a useful test on the efficiency of oral hygiene procedures. During the early period of instruction plaque should be stained before brushing. However, when the patient becomes experienced in oral hygiene techniques, he can occasionally use a disclosing agent after brushing to check the efficiency of his efforts.*

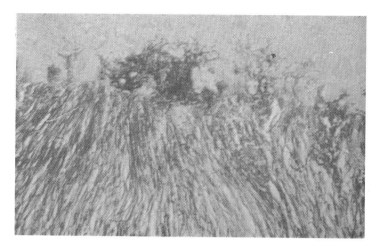

Figure 29. *Histological appearance of plaque using a simple staining technique after removing the sample from a tooth surface with a dental instrument. The filamentous nature of plaque can be seen.*

First, the patient should disclose plaque before toothbrushing. When he feels that he is experienced in oral hygiene procedures, he may use a disclosing tablet after toothbrushing (Figure 28) to check the efficacy of his technique.

Another method that can be used to help motivate patients is the microscopic demonstration of plaque bacteria and matrix by the dentist or hygienist, in samples taken from the patient's mouth. This can be an efficient adjunct in a plaque control regimen. This need not involve much expense because several inexpensive, but effective, microscopes are now available. The use of a simplified staining technique involving the use of crystal violet dye can show plaque within minutes of taking the sample (Figure 29).

Suggested Techniques

1. Take plaque sample by gently scraping a flat plastic dental instrument around the lingual aspect of a lower molar tooth.

2. Transfer scraping to a microscope slide. Spread out the sample otherwise it will appear as a solid mass. One drop of water often

41

helps in teasing or smearing the sample over the slide.

3. Pass the underside of the glass slide through a small flame for several seconds to fix the specimen.

4. Place one drop of crystal violet dye on to the specimen and leave for 60 seconds.

5. Wash off with tap water, dry with blotting paper and the specimen is ready for microscopic examination.

6. Place slide on microscope table and focus on specimen with a low power objective lens ($\times 5$ or $\times 10$).

7. Place one drop of immersion oil on the slide, over the stained specimen.

8. Gently rotate the oil-immersion objective lens into place and focus using the fine adjustment control.

Frequency of Brushing

Patients should be instructed to brush their teeth twice a day—in the morning after breakfast and in the evening before going to bed. However, it is far better that the patient cleans his teeth once a day thoroughly rather than in a quick and inefficient manner after every meal. If a once-a-day regimen is to be used the brushing period should be in the evening before going to bed. If a patient is willing to brush on more occasions, they should be related to meal times. Even in these cases, the brushing session in the evening should be the one which is carried out more efficiently, because the patient usually has more time than during an average day.

The Toothbrush

Toothbrushes should be replaced frequently because most adults and children use brushes that are no longer efficient. The average life of a toothbrush is about three months. The most popular type of brush has a straight, semirigid handle about six inches long, with a small head about one inch long (Figure 21). The bristles are about half an inch long and the tufts of bristles are trimmed to uniform height. For children, smaller brushes are advisable. Today most bristles are made of nylon. The stiffness of the nylon filaments depends upon the diameter and length of the filament. A brush made of 0.01 inch diameter (250 μm) filaments is considered a 'soft' brush; 0.012 inch (300 μm) a 'medium' brush; 0.014 inch (350 μm) a 'stiff' (hard) brush and 0.016 inch (400 μm) an 'extra stiff' (extra hard) brush. It has been shown that the end of the bristles is not important; round-end bristles do not appear to be any safer than cut-end bristles. It is well to recommend a 'medium' bristle brush because it cleans adequately. Patients with delicate or diseased gingival tissues should use a 'soft' toothbrush and a careful technique until the tissues return to normal (Hine 1956). The type of toothbrush used depends on the patient's preference. Studies of brush design have not revealed any superior type.

Methods of Brushing

1. Scrub method. This is carried out using a horizontal scrubbing motion with the bristles perpendicular to the surface of the teeth.

2. Fones technique. The teeth are held in occlusion and the brush is pressed vigorously against the teeth and gums, and revolved in circles with as large a diameter as possible.

3. Roll technique. This is performed by rotating the bristles from the gingiva to the occlusal edges of the teeth.

4. Vibratory or Bass techniques. These are designed to clean interproximal areas. The sides of the bristles are used for gingival massage, with bristles bent to prevent the ends from injuring the soft tissue. They are time-consuming, difficult to learn, and if improperly used can damage the gingiva.

a) Charters' technique. The brush is placed with the bristles at an angle of 45 degrees to the plane of occlusion, with the bristles pointed occlusally. Pressure is applied to the brush in a lateral and apical direction and the brush is vibrated rapidly a millimetre or so. The brush is reapplied three or four times in each embrasure.

b) Stillman's technique. The brush is parallel to the long axis of the tooth, with the bristles pointed apically and the ends of the bristles at the level of the gingival margin. Lateral pressure is applied to the brush, with vibration mesiodistally to force the bristles into the interproximal area. The brush is repeatedly applied to each embrasure.

5. 'Physiologic' technique. Using a very soft brush, clean from crown to gingiva with a gentle, sweeping motion.

Relative Merits of the Various Toothbrushing Techniques

Although the roll method of brushing teeth is widely advised, evidence to support its effectiveness is not readily found. Kimmelmann and Tassman (1960), Starkey (1961), McClure (1966), and Sangnes et al. (1972) have reported that in children, the scrubbing method is better than the roll method for dislodging debris from all surfaces. In addition it is suggested that the arch form and tooth form in the deciduous dentition are well suited to horizontal scrubbing strokes. It is unlikely that the gingiva will be damaged using such a technique.

A similar finding that a scrubbing technique is more effective than the roll technique in adults has been reported (Frandsen et al. 1970). They found that a scrubbing technique removed plaque as completely as did the Charters' technique, and did so much more rapidly. The scrub method cleaned as well in two minutes as the Charters' technique did in eight minutes, and cleaned better than the roll method, which took five minutes. With the latter two methods, much of the time required is spent in correct placement and positioning of the brush rather than in actual cleaning.

Children under seven years of age are not able to master an effective toothbrush technique, so it is essential to have a parent carry out the brushing (McClure 1966). A technique has been described by Starkey (1961) whereby the child leans the head back against the parent. The parent uses one forearm to cradle the head for support and uses the fingers of the same hand to retract the lips. The other hand is then free to carry out the brushing. Looking over the child gives a direct view of the teeth which can be cleaned using a scrubbing action on all surfaces (Figure 30).

Löe (1970) reported Charters' technique to be particularly effective for plaque removal. Although this method was designed specifically for cleaning between the teeth, Löe reported that the buccal and lingual surfaces were also cleaned adequately during this procedure. Although seven different methods of brushing were evaluated at the World Workshop in Periodontics (Ramfjord et al. 1966), the participants could not finally recommend any

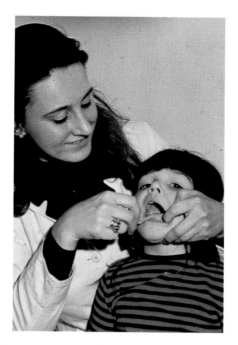

Figure 30. *The correct method for cleaning a child's teeth. The adult has good control over the child's head and can see the teeth during the cleaning routine.*

method as being superior to others in the removal of plaque. They concluded that the conscientious and correct application of a brushing technique was more effective and important than the technique.

Many studies carried out on the effectiveness of electric toothbrushes have come to the conclusion that they can be used just as efficiently as manual ones. Their use is especially indicated for the handicapped patient. Battery operated models become less efficient with loss of power because of infrequent changing of the batteries.

Dental Flossing

No matter how efficiently one uses a toothbrush, plaque will not be

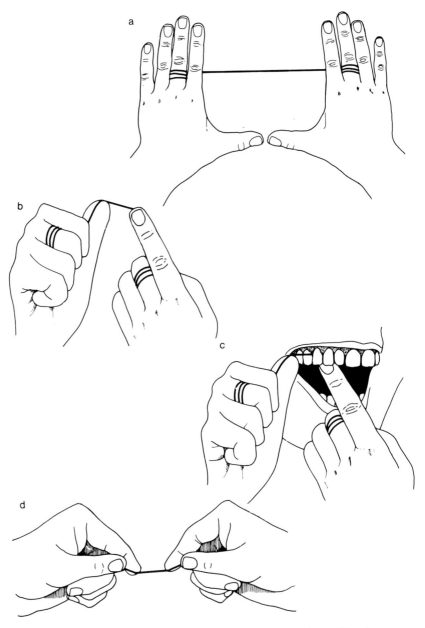

Figure 31. *(a) (b) (c) and (d) Technique for the effective use of dental floss.*

removed between the teeth. During oral hygiene instruction the patient must be introduced to dental floss. It must be pointed out that the use of dental floss is the only decisive way of removing plaque from interproximal regions. The effect of flossing in reducing the incidence of dental caries on interproximal surfaces was reported in a 20-month study of 88 six-year-old children (Wright et al. 1977). The flossed surfaces were found to have 53 per cent fewer cavities than control surfaces. Axelsson and Lindhe (1975) demonstrated almost total caries inhibition in children on a regimen of frequent plaque control, fluoride treatment and oral hygiene instruction. The data emphasized the importance of plaque removal and oral hygiene for caries prevention. Because flossing requires a reasonable degree of dexterity, the patient must be taught the correct technique and told to practice daily. There are a number of plastic floss applicators available but it is doubtful whether they offer any advantage over the conventional hand techniques. There are two main techniques. In the first, a length of floss about 24 inches is cut off. The ends of the floss are lightly wrapped around the middle fingers of both hands (Figure 31a). To clean between the upper right posterior teeth pass the floss over the right thumb and the forefinger of the left hand (Figure 31b). The thumb is held to the buccal aspects of the teeth and helps in retracting the cheek (Figure 31c). To clean between the teeth in the upper left quadrant, pass the floss over the left thumb and the forefinger of the right hand. Now the left thumb is on the buccal aspects of the teeth and the right forefinger is on the palatal aspect. To clean the interproximal regions of all lower teeth, hold the floss with the forefingers of both hands (Figure 31d). It will be possible to insert the floss gently between all lower teeth with the floss over the forefingers in this position.

In the second method a loop is formed having a diameter of about four inches. The fingers of both hands are placed within the loop so that the finger or thumb tips used to place the floss between the teeth will be only about half an inch apart.

Suggestions for Flossing

1. The fingers controlling the floss should not be more than half an inch apart.

2. Do not force the floss between the teeth. Insert it gently by sawing it back and forth at the contact point. Allow it to slide gently into place.

3. Using both fingers move the floss up and down about six times on the approximal surface of one tooth, and then using a see-saw action, draw it back and forth along the interproximal surface. Repeat on the approximal surface of the adjacent tooth.

4. It is important to ensure that the floss be wrapped around the interproximal surface of each tooth in turn within any one space.

5. When the interproximal surfaces are clean they often make a squeaking noise when the floss is moved over the surface.

6. Loosened debris should be removed by rinsing the mouth vigorously with water.

7. Pass floss carefully into the subgingival region so as not to damage the soft tissue.

8. After each molar interproximal area is cleaned, a length of clean floss is brought into play by winding a turn on to the middle finger of one hand and off the middle finger of the other hand. Alternatively, if the loop technique is used, a length of clean floss is prepared by moving the fingers around the loop. Dental floss can

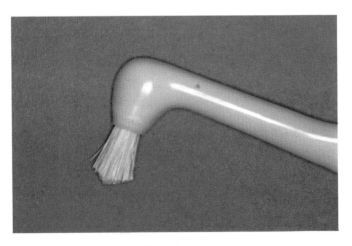

Figure 32. *An interspace brush.*

48

be obtained in either a waxed or unwaxed variety. A number of workers feel that the most suitable floss is that which consists of a large number of unwaxed microscopic nylon filaments having a minimum of twist. Because unwaxed floss must be used in the initial cleaning regimen before topical fluoride therapy, it may not be necessary to stock waxed floss in the dental office. To be of any value dental floss must be used systematically as already outlined.

In addition to obtaining floss in dispensers suitable for use in the dental office, small reels of unwaxed floss containing about 50 yards are available. These can be carried by patients in a handbag or small pocket, and are therefore suitable for daily use. With older children, flossing should also be included in the oral hygiene routine even if it is at first confined to the mesial and distal interproximal surfaces of the first permanent molars.

Oral Rinsing

The use of toothbrushing and dental floss will loosen many particles of food, plaque and debris. Their further removal will be aided by vigorous rinsing of the mouth using water. The same procedure will do much to speed the oral clearance of semi-fluid carbohydrates. After snacks and meals when it is not possible to use a toothbrush rinsing with water should be recommended. A technique should be adopted that attempts to force water between the teeth by vigorous blowing and sucking actions with the mouth closed. Such a rinsing procedure may be carried out using a dilute fluoride solution where it will have a specific caries preventive effect.

Other Devices

Because of its single tuft, an interspace brush (Figure 32) can be manoeuvred relatively easily into otherwise inaccessible regions. Such brushes are particularly useful if the patient has crown or bridgework, which are usually very difficult to keep thoroughly clean. Wood sticks for interproximal cleaning are readily obtainable and can be a useful aid to oral hygiene. They were originally

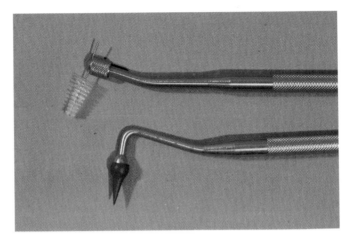

Figure 33. *Examples of interdental stimulators.*

devised for gingival massage but, because the susceptible area, the crevicular epithelium, is not subject to keratinization, it seems that their beneficial effect is plaque removal. If wood sticks are used, care should be taken in their use because breakage and retention of the pieces can be painful.

Interdental stimulators (Figure 33) can be used to massage the tissue between the teeth and help to reduce local oedema. Stimulators should be placed at right angles to the tissue to reach the col depression. However, indiscriminate use of this approach may blunt the papilla, with an unattractive and potentially damaging result.

The use of water irrigation devices reduces bacterial loads and cellular debris, but does not remove plaque efficiently. They can be useful in the removal of soft oral debris in relation to bridgework. They should therefore be used as adjuncts rather than as primary therapeutic instruments.

Chemical Plaque Control

Much research has been carried out in recent years in the use of agents which might inhibit the deposition of dental plaque.

Several antibiotics show plaque-reducing properties and some can inhibit plaque formation completely. Impressive results have also been obtained using topical chlorhexidine to prevent the initial formation of plaque. However, long-term effects of changing the oral flora must be evaluated before any of these methods can be considered as a practical solution to the problem of lifelong plaque control. Use of combinations of minor antibiotics, which have little importance in systemic chemotherapy, may be one answer to plaque control (Bowen 1977, pers. comm.).

The production of dextrans by oral streptococci has been implicated in the formation of 'sticky' gelatinous plaques. In animal experiments, dextranase will help to disperse such plaques. However, it is unlikely that a single enzyme, or even combinations of enzymes, could be an efficient plaque remover in man.

Topically applied fluorides may have an effect as a plaque-preventive agent by reducing the ability of the enamel surface to adsorb protein.

Vaccination

Bowen (1969b) showed that monkeys vaccinated with whole, live dextran-forming streptococci developed substantially fewer carious lesions than control unvaccinated animals. A series of experiments carried out over a three- to seven-year period demonstrated a significant degree of caries prevention in monkeys inoculated with *Streptococcus mutans* and maintained on a caries-promoting diet (Bowen et al. 1975). Preparations of whole cells or broken cells were most successful and experiments indicated that intraoral submucosal injection was more likely to be effective than subcutaneous injection. Further work by this group has shown the great potential of this method for caries prevention.

Diet

In theory dental caries could be prevented by removing dietary sucrose or other fermentable carbohydrates from the diet. However, this approach is impractical because it is difficult, if not impossible, to change a nation's diet. The object of dietary counselling is to provide the patient with a realistic and acceptable diet (see Chapter 8).

References

Axelsson, P. and Lindhe, J., *Commun. Dent. Oral Epidemiol.*, 1975, **3**, 156.

Bowen, W. H., International Conference on Dental Plaque, Am. Dent. Assoc. & Warner-Lambert Pharm. Co., New Jersey, USA, 1969a.

Bowen, W. H., *Br. Dent. J.*, 1969b, **126**, 159.

Bowen, W. H., Cohen, B., Cole, M. F. and Colman, G., *Br. Dent. J.*, 1975, **139**, 45.

Brilliant, H., US Patent Office, US Patent No. 3–309–274, 1967.

Frandsen, A. M., Barbano, J. P., Somi, J. D., Chang, J. J. and Burke, A. D., *Scand. J. Dent. Res.*, 1970, **78**, 459.

Greene, J. C. and Vermillion, J. R., *J. Dent. Res.*, 1971, **50**, 184.

Hefferren, H., Cooley, R. O., Hall, J. B., Olsen, N. H. and Lyon, H. W., *J. Am. Dent. Assoc.*, 1971, **82**, 1353.

Hine, M. K., *Int. Dent. J.*, 1956, **6**, 15.

Kimmelmann, B. B. and Tassman, G. C., *J. Dent. Child.*, 1960, **27**, 60.

Lang, N. P., Oftrgaard, E. and Löe, H., *J. Periodont. Res.*, 1972, **7**, 59.

Löe, H., *Dental Plaque*, W. McHugh (Ed.), E. & S. Livingstone, Edinburgh and London, 1970.

Löe, H., Theilade, E. and Jensen, S. B., *J. Periodont.*, 1965, **36**, 177.

McClure, D. B., *J. Dent. Child.*, 1966, **33**, 205.

Ramfjord, S. P., Kerr, D. A. and Ash, M. A., *Edits of World Workshop in Periodontics*, Ann Arbour, The University of Michigan, USA, 1966.

Sangnes, G., Zachrisson, B. and Gjermo, P., *J. Dent. Child.*, 1972, **34**, 94.

Sheiham, A., *Dent. Practit. Dent. Rec.*, 1969, **19**, 232.

Sheiham, A., *Dent. Health*, 1971, **10**, 1.

Starkey, P., *J. Dent. Child.*, 1961, **18**, 42.

Wright, G. Z., Banting, D. W. and Feasby, W. H., *J. Dent. Res.*, 1977, **56**, 574.

4. Topical Fluorides: Development and Clinical Trials

The aim of topical fluoride therapy is the deposition of fluoride into the surface layer of tooth enamel to form fluorapatite, so as to decrease the caries susceptibility of the tissue.

$$Ca_{10}(PO_4)_6(OH)_2 + 2F^- \rightarrow Ca_{10}(PO_4)_6F_2 + 2OH^-$$

enamel hydroxyapatite + fluoride   fluorapatite + hydroxyl

Mechanisms whereby fluoride reduces caries are complex, but may be summarized under the following headings.

1. By rendering enamel more resistant to acid dissolution. Under the influence of fluoride:

a) Larger enamel crystals are formed with fewer imperfections. This stabilizes the lattice and presents a smaller surface area per unit volume for dissolution.

b) Enamel has a lower carbonate content, thus giving reduced solubility.

c) Reprecipitation of calcium phosphates occurs and fluoride favours their crystallization as apatite.

It is claimed that the initial rate of dissolution of hydroxyapatite is the same as fluorapatite (Gray et al. 1962). However, the subsequent formation of secondary precipitates (such as calcium fluoride) on the surface of the enamel crystals reduces the rate of diffusion of hydrogen ions and of undissociated acid to the crystals, thus reducing their rate of solution.

2. By inhibiting bacterial enzyme systems which convert

sugars into acids in plaque. For this to occur, fluoride must be present as free ionic fluoride and not be bound up in plaque (Jenkins 1967).

3. By inhibiting storage of intracellular polysaccharides. In this way the accumulation of carbohydrate within the cell is prevented. This could otherwise be used to form acids between meals.

4. At high concentration fluoride is toxic to bacteria. Certain species may therefore be eliminated for short periods after topical fluoride therapy. However, this is obviously only a temporary benefit of topical fluoride therapy.

5. By reducing the tendency of the enamel surface to adsorb proteins. Several in vitro reports have shown that plaque does not build up so readily on enamel surfaces treated with fluoride. This may be because fluoride reduces the surface energy of the teeth (Glantz 1969) and the tendency of the enamel surface to adsorb proteins (Ericson and Ericsson 1967).

Clinical trials have failed to demonstrate any plaque-reducing effect. However, a recent pilot study on humans demonstrated a significant reduction in plaque in fluoride-treated quadrants relative to controls after topical application of a fluoride gel (Pearlman and Joyston-Bechal 1973).

6. Modification in size and shape of teeth. Animal experiments have suggested that fluoride intake during tooth development may reduce the size of teeth and produce more rounded cusps and shallower fissures. Such observations have been recorded in humans from high-fluoride areas in the UK (Forrest 1956). However, the scientific basis for this is poor.

7. Remineralization. Fluoride favours precipitation of calcium and phosphate ions in the form of apatite rather than as soluble calcium phosphates (McCann and Brudevold 1966). Experiments on remineralization of carious human enamel in vitro have shown that the presence of low concentrations of fluoride greatly enhances the reprecipitation of mineral ions into the damaged enamel (Silverstone 1972).

Fluoride Agents

Sodium Fluoride

Bibby (1942) was the first to use fluoride solutions on teeth in the dental office as a caries-preventive measure. He reported that applications of 0.1 per cent sodium fluoride, three times a year, produced a 33 per cent reduction in caries experience in children from 10 to 13 years of age. In this study, on 78 children, the solution was applied to half the mouth, the untreated half acting as a control.

Sodium fluoride was selected on the basis that it was a soluble salt and was employed in artificial fluoridation of water supplies. After this, research was concentrated on finding the optimum concentration and the most effective technique. This led to the classical studies reported by Knutson (1948) in which a two per cent solution was used.

Technique

1. Tooth crowns were cleaned using a rubber cup and prophylaxis paste.

2. A two per cent solution was applied to teeth in an isolated and dried quadrant, or to half the mouth.

3. Teeth were allowed to remain moist with the solution for three to four minutes.

4. Application was repeated on the other quadrants.

5. Second, third and fourth applications' not preceded by prophylaxis, were given at intervals of about one week.

6. Treatments were recommended at three, seven, 11 and 13 years of age to coincide with eruption of new teeth.

Reductions in caries were reported as 30 to 40 per cent among children living in low fluoride areas.

Further studies by other workers confirmed the preventive properties of topically applied sodium fluoride. According to Horowitz and Heifetz (1970), certain aspects of its potential usefulness need further investigation, though these questions also apply to other agents. However:

1. Further long-term studies must be carried out to determine precisely how long after treatment a topical agent continues to exert a beneficial effect.

2. Some investigations suggest that a fall-off in effectiveness may occur in less than three years (Syrrist and Karlsen 1954).

3. Optimum frequency of application remains to be determined.

Advantages of Sodium Fluoride

1. It is stable chemically when stored in plastic or polythene containers.

2. It has an acceptable taste.

3. The solution is non-irritating to the gingiva.

4. It does not cause discolouration of the teeth.

Disadvantage

With the Knutson technique, the patient must make four visits within a relatively short time.

Stannous Fluoride

Because of the time-consuming regimen described by Knutson (1948), further laboratory studies were undertaken.

Of the compounds tested, stannous fluoride (SnF_2) was shown by Muhler and his co-workers (1950) to be more effective in reducing the rate of dissolution of enamel by acid in vitro. Howell et al. (1955) compared the efficacy of two per cent SnF_2 and two per cent NaF when applied according to Knutson's technique. Stannous fluoride proved more efficient than sodium fluoride, reductions being 59 per cent and 30 per cent, respectively. Subsequent studies by Slack (1956), Nevitt et al. (1958) and Gish et al. (1959) confirmed the effectiveness of two per cent SnF_2.

However, the reductions reported were far less than those recorded by Howell and his co-workers (1955). Jordan et al. (1959) and Gish et al. (1959) reported that annual applications of eight per cent SnF_2 produced significant caries reductions. This single regimen was more desirable than the much longer technique advocated by Knutson.

56

Technique

1. Rubber-cup prophylaxis; tooth surfaces cleaned and polished with pumice for five to ten seconds each (the pumice carried between contact points using unwaxed dental floss).

2. Either a quadrant or half the mouth is isolated and dried.

3. A freshly prepared eight per cent solution of SnF_2 is applied continuously to the teeth with cotton applicators so that the enamel surfaces are kept moist with it for four minutes. Reapplication is usually required every 15 to 30 seconds.

In highly susceptible patients, the topical application should be repeated at least once every six months; for those not particularly caries-prone, a single treatment can be given once a year. Mercer and Muhler (1961) showed that a second application of eight per cent SnF_2 given within a few days provided no additional preventive effect.

Much of the work dealing with SnF_2 as a topical fluoride agent has been conducted by Muhler and his associates at the University of Indiana, USA. They have reported on many occasions that annual or six-monthly applications of an eight per cent solution of SnF_2 produce a significant decrease in development of new carious lesions (Muhler 1958), and their trials indicate benefits exceeding the 30 to 40 per cent reductions generally accepted for two per cent NaF. Levels of prevention ranging from 47 to 78 per cent on new DMF surfaces have been recorded.

Other investigators have found SnF_2 effective, although usually to a lesser extent than that reported by Muhler et al. Peterson and Williamson (1962) reported a 26 per cent lower increment in DMF teeth after two annual applications of eight per cent SnF_2 solution. Law et al. (1961) found that a single application produced a reduction of about 17 per cent in development of new carious teeth after one year and Harris (1963) that six-monthly treatments led to a 23 per cent reduction in new lesions.

However, in conflict with many favourable reports, a few more recent studies using SnF_2 have shown extremely disappointing results. Wellock et al. (1965), found that in the case of children it failed to yield any reductions after one year. Negative results were also obtained in Sweden by Torell and Ericsson (1965) in a two-year study: no benefit was observed in a group of children after two annual applications of a 10 per cent SnF_2 solution, while Horowitz and Lucye (1966) similarly found no preventive effect in children who received a topical application of eight per cent SnF_2 annually for two years, after either the first or second year.

Disadvantages of Stannous Fluoride

1. It is not stable in aqueous solution, undergoes fairly rapid hydrolysis and oxidation, and forms stannous hydroxide and the stannic ion. This reaction reduces its effectiveness, and consequently a fresh solution must be used each time.

2. Because an eight per cent solution of SnF_2 is astringent and disagreeable in taste, its application is unpleasant (Horowitz and Heifetz 1970). Unfortunately the addition of flavouring agents is contraindicated.

3. The solution sometimes causes a reversible tissue irritation, shown by gingival blanching. This reaction usually occurs in patients with poor gingival health.

4. Pigmentation and staining of teeth after SnF_2 has been reported by many. It usually appears in association with carious lesions, hypocalcified areas of enamel, and around the margins of restorations. Backer-Dirks (1961) estimated that 95 per cent of children had pigmented teeth after SnF_2 application and Wellock et al. (1965) reported staining in 60 per cent.

5. Because SnF_2 produces staining it is difficult to measure caries in test and control groups. Enamel lesions can be masked clinically, photographically and by radiography (Glass, 1967; Lobene et al. 1966). This may lead to errors in diagnosis and be responsible for many so-called 'reversals' reported in SnF_2 studies (Forrester and Auger 1971).

Acidulated Phosphate Fluoride (APF)

Brudevold and his co-workers (1963) reported laboratory studies showing that an APF solution produced an increased uptake of fluoride by enamel compared with either stannous fluoride or neutral sodium fluoride.

The success of a topical fluoride agent depends largely on the extent to which it is capable of depositing fluoride in the enamel as fluorapatite. An ideal one would react with enamel to form maximal amounts of fluorapatite quickly. Water fluoridation forms fluorapatite in the enamel, in terms of months or years, whereas a topical solution must react in minutes.

The crystalline structure of enamel is made more stable by acquisition of fluoride according to the following reaction:

$$Ca_{10}(PO_4)_6(OH)_2 + 2F^- \leftrightharpoons Ca_{10}(PO_4)_6F_2 + 2OH^-$$
enamel hydroxyopatite + fluoride　　fluorapatite + hydroxyl

Fluoride competes with, and displaces, the hydroxyl groups of the hydroxyapatite molecule to form fluorapatite. This reaction may be speeded up by:

1. Raising the concentration of fluoride in solution.

2. Lowering the pH, thus making the solution more acid.

However, both methods may produce undesirable side-effects:

1. Increasing fluoride concentration may cause the following:

$$Ca_{10}(PO_4)_6(OH)_2 + 20F^- \leftrightharpoons 10CaF_2 + 6PO_4^- + 2OH^-$$
enamel hydroxyapatite + high　　calcium fluoride + phosphate
concentration of fluoride　　　　　+ hydroxyl

Calcium fluoride has a different crystal structure from apatite and its formation is associated with decomposition of the mineral phase of enamel.

2. Lowering the pH. It is accepted that enamel in the presence of acid may break down according to the following reaction:

$$Ca_{10}(PO_4)_6(OH)_2 + 8H^+ \leftrightharpoons 10Ca^{++} + 6HPO_4^- + H_2O$$
enamel hydroxyapatite + acid　　calcium + phosphate + water

Thus, increased fluoride could be deposited into enamel only if both calcium fluoride formation, and demineralization, could be suppressed. Brudevold noticed that both these unfavourable reactions resulted in phosphate as a breakdown product. He reasoned that since the reactions are reversible, introduction of phosphate into the solution containing high fluoride at low pH would suppress the undesirable effects because of a shift in equilibrium of the reactions from left to right, yielding intact hydroxyapatite as the principal reaction product. Therefore, if enamel is brought into contact with high concentrations of fluoride at low pH, in the presence of phosphate, rapid fluoride deposition should occur with no significant enamel breakdown.

Clinical Studies

Initial clinical studies on topically applied acidulated phosphate fluoride solutions gave excellent results. After two years of annual applications children showed a 67 per cent smaller increment in DMF teeth and a 70 per cent reduction in DMF surfaces, compared with untreated controls (Wellock and Brudevold 1963). When a two per cent solution of sodium fluoride was applied to half the mouth, and a two per cent sodium fluoride solution acidified with orthophosphoric acid (APF) to the other half, it was found that the half treated with the acid phosphate had about 50 per cent fewer new carious lesions than that treated with neutral sodium fluoride, the difference being highly significant (Parmeijer et al. 1963).

The preventive effects shown in more recent studies have tended to be smaller than those obtained initially, but are nevertheless encouraging. Wellock et al. (1965) reported that after two annual applications of APF children had 44 per cent fewer new DMF teeth and 52 per cent fewer new DMF surfaces compared with untreated controls. Cartwright et al. (1968) obtained a 49 per cent reduction in DMF teeth after two years in children who received the topical application at six-monthly intervals. Horowitz (1968, 1969) showed that three years after receiving annual applications of APF, children had 28 per cent fewer new DMF surfaces compared with controls and 41 per cent fewer DMF surfaces following APF solution at six-monthly intervals.

Technique

The technique for application of APF solution is similar to that for other fluoride agents. The crowns of teeth are cleaned with prophylaxis paste using a rubber cup, and unwaxed dental floss is

60

employed to carry the paste between interstitial contact regions. The solution is then applied to a dried and isolated quadrant, or half the mouth, enamel surfaces remaining moist for four minutes.

Advantages of APF

1. It is chemically stable when stored in plastic or polythene containers.

2. It has a tolerable taste (and can be flavoured without upsetting the fluoride content).

3. It will not stain enamel surfaces or pellicle.

4. It is not astringent to gingival tissues.

5. Clinical trials have shown it to be an effective caries preventive agent.

6. Laboratory studies have established that enamel takes up significantly more fluoride from APF than from other fluoride agents.

APF Gels

Relatively few studies have been carried out on the use of APF gels. Application in wax trays produced a 24 per cent reduction in DMF surfaces after three years compared with controls (Horowitz 1968; 1969). Bryan and Williams (1968) found after one year 28 per cent fewer new DMF surfaces among children eight to 12 years of age after a single treatment with APF gel in foam-rubber trays, and Ingraham and Williams (1970) found a 41 per cent reduction over two years. Use of an APF solution over a similar time-span yielded non-significant reductions.

In a study by Cons et al. (1970), test groups received either APF gel, APF solution, neutral sodium fluoride or stannous fluoride. After three years significant reductions were found only in the case of APF gel. Supervised self-application of fluoride gels in polyvinyl mouthpieces was tested at Cheektowaga, New York (Englander et al. 1967). Children used it for six minutes each school day for two years. At the end of 21 months reductions of 75 per cent and 80 per cent in new DMF surfaces among two groups were recorded.

The clinical advantage of using gels is that the whole mouth can be treated at once rather than separate quadrants by solution technique, but since gels are viscous, poorly fitting trays or mouth-pieces may apply them only to freely exposed buccal, lingual and occlusal surfaces. Moreover, to be effective against smooth surface caries, the gel must penetrate the interstitial regions. Since gels must be used in trays the design of these is of extreme importance: variations in results of trials could well be related to this factor.

In addition to the clinical advantage of treating the whole mouth at once, gels have another important advantage. Substantial amounts of fluoride are deposited into enamel from topical treat-ments but most of it soon leaches away into the oral environment (Brudevold et al. 1967; Mellberg et al. 1966). Laboratory experiments indicate that this loss is essentially complete within 24 hours. If fluoride ions can be 'trapped' at the enamel surface for longer periods, this could result in a greater uptake by enamel.

Several workers have shown an increase in enamel fluoride in vitro after application of coating materials to the enamel (Brudevold et al. 1966; Mellberg et al. 1967). Fluoride gels also exhibit a somewhat similar mechanism, a thin layer remaining on enamel surfaces acting as a fluoride ion reservoir. A significant increase in fluoride content of surface enamel has been shown four and 60 days after a gel (Hotz 1972), and higher levels of fluoride were deposited from gel than from APF solution (Clarkson 1972). In addition, APF gel was more effective in preventing artificial caries than either an APF solution or other topical fluoride agents (Clarkson and Silverstone 1974).

Therefore, it is evident that fluoride gels have great potential as caries preventive agents, provided that the problems are borne in mind.

Comparison of Methods

A study in the USA provided an example (Table 2) of how much can be achieved by spending a given amount of money on different methods of fluoridation, and also compared the number of cavities which could be treated for the same sum (Gish 1968).

Water fluoridation has by far the lowest cost per cavity. How-ever, topical fluorides can be seen to be effective, not only in children but also in young adults. Teeth should preferably be

Table 2. Comparative results per $100,000 spent.

	Cavities prevented
1. Water fluoridation	666,660
2. Self-applied fluorides	233,330
3. Topical fluorides	60,000
4. Fluoride dentifrices	25,600
5. Dental restorations	16,666 cavities restored

treated as soon after eruption as possible, since these benefit most from topical fluoride therapy (Averill et al. 1967; Horowitz and Heifetz 1969).

It would be reasonable to expect some benefit in adults of all ages, although clinical trials in this area are limited and conflicting (Klinkerberg and Bibby 1950; Kulter and Ireland 1953; Rickles and Becks 1951). Benefits might be expected in prevention of recurrent caries around existing restorations rather than in prevention of initial lesions as in children and young adults.

Recent evidence has also shown that topical fluorides can give additional caries prevention even in areas receiving fluoridated drinking water (Englander et al. 1971).

In subsequent chapters fluoride agents, systems and devices currently available will be discussed critically and details of a recommended topical fluoride regimen will be given.

References

Averill, H. M., Averill, J. E. and Ritz, A. G., *J. Am. Dent. Assoc.*, 1967, **74**, 997.

Backer-Dirks, O., *Caries Prevention by Fluorine-containing Dentifrices*, **37**, 1961.

Bibby, B. G., *J. Dent Res.*, 1942, **21**, 314.

Brudevold, F., DePaola, P. F., Quinn, K. and Kelly, K., Abst. No. 218, Iadr, Miami, USA, 1966.

Brudevold, F., McCann, H. G., Nilsson, R., Richardson, B. and Coklica, V., *J. Dent Res.*, 1967, **46**, 37.

Brudevold, F., Savory, A., Gardner, D. E., Spinelli, M. and Speirs, R., *Arch. Oral Biol.*, 1963, **8**, 167.

Preventive Dentistry

Bryan, E. T. and Williams, J. E., *J. Pub. Health Dent.*, 1968, **28**, 182.

Cartwright, H. V., Lindahl, R. L. and Bawden, J. W., *J. Dent. Child.*, 1968, **35**, 36.

Clarkson, B. H., *J. Dent. Res.*, 1972, **51**, 1262.

Clarkson, B. H. and Silverstone, L. M., *J. Int. Assoc. Dent. Child.*, 1974, **5**, 27.

Cons, N. C., Janerich, D. T. and Sennings, R. S., *J. Am. Dent. Assoc.*, 1970, **80**, 777.

Englander, H. R., Keyes, P. H., Gestwicki, M. and Sutz, H. A., *J. Am. Dent. Assoc.*, 1967, **75**, 638.

Englander, H. R., Sherrill, L. T., Miller, B. G., Carlos, J. T., Mellberg, J. R. and Senning, R. S., *J. Am. Dent. Assoc.*, 1971, **82**, 354.

Ericson, T. and Ericsson, Y., *Helv. Odont. Acta*, 1967, **11**, 10.

Forrest, J. R., *Br. Dent. J.*, 1956, **100**, 195.

Forrester, D. J. and Auger, M. F., *J. Dent. Child.*, 1971, **39**, 272.

Gish, C. W., *Am. Dent. Assoc. Newsletter*, 1968, **21**, 23.

Gish, C. W., Howell, C. L., and Muhler, J. C., *J. Dent. Child.*, 1959, **26**, 300.

Glantz, P., *Odont. Revy*, 1969, **20**, 17.

Glass, R. L., *Arch. Oral Biol.*, 1967, **12**, 401.

Gray, J. A., Francis, M. D. and Griebstein, W. J., *Chemistry and Prevention of Dental Caries*, Thomas, Illinois, 1962.

Harris, R., *Aust. Dent. J.*, 1963, **8**, 335.

Horowitz, H. S., *J. Oral Ther.*, 1968, **4**, 286.

Horowitz, H. S., *J. Am. Dent. Assoc.*, 1969, **78**, 568.

Horowitz, H. S. and Heifetz, S. B., *J. Dent. Child.*, 1969, **36**, 335.

Horowitz, H. S. and Heifetz, S. B., *J. Am. Dent. Assoc.*, 1970, **81**, 166.

Horowitz, H. S. and Lucye, H. S., *J. Oral Ther.*, 1966, **3**, 17.

Hotz, P., *Helv. Odont. Acta*, 1972, **16**, 32.

Howell, C. H., Gish, C. W., Smiley, R. D. and Muhler, J. C., *J. Am. Dent. Assoc.*, 1955, **50**. 14.

Ingraham, R. Q. and Williams, J. E., *J. Tenn. Dent Assoc.*, 1970, **50**, 5.

Jenkins, G. N., *Int. Dent. J.*, 1967, **17**, 552.

Jordan, W. A., Snyder, J. R. and Wilson, V., *J. Dent. Child.*, 1959, **26**, 355.

Klinkerberg, E. and Bibby, B. G., *J. Dent. Res.*, 1950, **29**, 4.

Knutson, J. W., *J. Am. Dent. Assoc.*, 1948, **36**, 37.

Kulter, N. H. and Ireland, R. L., *J. Dent. Res.*, 1953, **32**, 458.

Law, F. E., Jeffries, M. H. and Sheary, H. C., *Pub. Health Rep.*, 1961, **76**, 287.

Lobene, R., Zulgar-Nam, B. and Hein, J., *J. Oral Ther.*, 1966, **3**, 35.

McCann, H. and Brudevold, E., *Environmental Variations in Oral Disease*, American Academy for the Advancement of Science, Washington, 1966.

Mellberg, J. R., Laakso, P. V. and Nicholson, C. R., *Arch. Oral Biol.*, 1966, **11**, 1213.

Mellberg, J. R., Nicholson, C. R. and Laakso, P. V., *Arch. Oral Biol.*, 1967, **12**, 1177.

Mercer, V. H. and Muhler, J. C., *J. Dent Child.*, 1961, **28**, 84.

Muhler, J. C., *J. Dent. Res.*, 1958, **37**, 415.

Muhler, J. C., Boyd, T. M. and Huysen, G., *J. Dent. Res.*, 1950, **29**, 182.

Nevitt, G. A., Witter, D. H. and Bowman, W. D., *Pub. Health Rep.*, 1958, **73**, 847.

Parmeijer, J. H. N., Hunt, E. E. and Brudevold, F., *Arch. Oral Biol.*, 1963, **8**, 179.

Pearlman, B. A. and Joyston-Bechal, S., *J. Dent. Res.*, 1973, **52**, 953.

Peterson, J. K. and Williamson, L., *Pub. Health Rep.*, 1962, **77**, 39.

Rickles, N. H. and Becks, H., *J. Dent. Res.*, 1951, **30**, 757.

Silverstone, L. M., *Proc. Roy. Soc. Med.*, 1972, **65**, 906.

Slack, G. L., *Br. Dent. J.*, 1956, **101**, 7.

Syrrist, A. and Karlsen, K., *Br. Dent. J.*, 1954, **97**, 1.

Torell, P. and Ericsson, Y., *Acta Odont. Scand.*, 1965, **23**, 287.

Wellock, W. D. and Brudevold, F., *Arch. Oral Biol.*, 1963, **8**, 179.

Wellock, W. D., Maitland, A. and Brudevold, F., *Arch. Oral Biol.*, 1965, **10**, 453.

5. Topical Fluorides: Clinical Techniques and Materials

Of the fluoride solutions available for topical application in the dental office, stannous fluoride and acidulated phosphate fluoride (APF) are the most popular.

Stannous Fluoride Solutions

Stannous fluoride is not stable in aqueous solution because it undergoes rapid hydrolysis and oxidation to form stannous hydroxide and the stannic ion. This reaction reduces its effectiveness and, as a result, a freshly prepared solution must be used each time.

An eight per cent solution is prepared by mixing 0.8 g of stannous fluoride salt with 10 ml of distilled water in the glass vessel provided, and shaking until the salt goes into solution. If the gingival tissues are damaged during prophylaxis, the application should be postponed. It has been shown (Swieterman et al. 1961) that injured or inflamed gingivae are affected adversely by stannous fluoride. Muhler (1957) also reported that mild blanching of the free gingival margins may occur in normal tissues. Although the astringent taste of stannous fluoride is disliked by many patients, flavouring agents should not be added to the topical agent because they may interfere with the mechanism of fluoride deposition.

After a rubber-cup prophylaxis, a quadrant of the mouth is isolated and dried. Freshly prepared eight per cent stannous fluoride solution is then applied to the clean, dried enamel surfaces, which are kept moistened with the solution for four minutes.

A 'cotton bud', or cotton wool wrapped around the end of an orange-wood stick, is used to apply the solution to enamel surfaces. The solution should also be taken into interproximal regions by gently passing unwaxed dental floss between these areas. The essential stages in the application technique, the advantages and disadvantages of stannous fluoride were discussed in Chapter 4.

Acidulated Phosphate Fluoride Solutions

Acidulated phosphate fluoride solution (APF) is used in a similar manner to stannous fluoride solution and to any other fluoride solution used for topical application. There are a number of different brands of APF solution available, but all are essentially similar in that they conform with the Brudevold formulation (Brudevold et al. 1963). This was discussed in some detail in Chapter 4. The APF solutions available differ mainly in the flavouring agents that are added. Some of the more exotic flavours (e.g. wild cherry, tropical fruit) are not as well accepted by children as the more conventional orange and lemon flavours. The main advantages of APF solution over stannous fluoride solution are its chemical stability when stored in plastic or polythene containers, and the fact that it does not stain enamel or pellicle, nor is it astringent to gingival tissues. Also, the addition of flavouring agents does not interfere with the mechanism of fluoride deposition.

Acidulated Phosphate Fluoride Gels

APF gels are more popular for clinical use than are solutions. One reason for this is that when used with application trays, either one arch or the whole mouth can be treated at the same time. In addition, the operator does not have to reapply the fluoride agent to the enamel during the exposure to keep enamel surfaces constantly moistened as with a solution. Moisture control is not a problem when the trays are seated in the mouth. Since their first introduction, many fluoride gels have appeared on the market. As with APF solutions, they are all very similar because they conform with the Brudevold formulation (Brudevold et al. 1963).

Fluoride gels are aqueous solutions of APF to which a water-soluble polymer, such as sodium carboxymethyl cellulose, has been added. This thickens the solution to a consistency where retention of the solution by the tooth is made easy. If fluoride ions can be 'trapped' at the enamel surface for longer periods, such as in the use of a fluoride gel, this results in a greater deposition of fluoride (Clarkson and Silverstone 1974). Recent studies have shown that most proprietary materials are not gels at all, because they exhibit

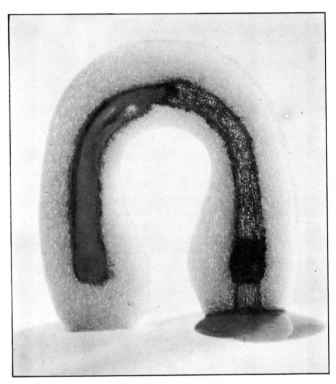

Figure 34. *A comparison between conventional APF gels and the new thixotropic gel. A conventional APF gel has been placed into the right-hand side of the application tray while the thixotropic gel was placed into the left-hand side. The conventional gel flows under gravity in contrast to the thixotropic gel which stays in situ and remains stationary under its own weight.*

no elastic effects (Braden 1974), but are mostly thixotropic solutions.

More recently, however, a new type of APF fluoride gel has been introduced. Whereas the conventional 'gels' are really viscous solutions, the new material is a thixotropic gel. When routine fluoride 'gels' are poured into an application tray they flow under gravity. However, the new thixotropic APF gel stays in situ and remains stationary under its own weight (Figure 34) in contrast with conventional gels which continue to flow. The fluoride concentration of this new gel (Gel II, Pacemaker Corp., Portland, Oregon, and AlphaGel, Amalgamated Dental, London) is the same as that in other APF gels; it is only the gelling agent that is different. Thus, when used with a suitable application tray, there will be a change in state—from gel to solution—at the interproximal region provided sufficient pressure is applied at that site.

This highlights the importance of using a well-fitting application tray. It should result in the material flowing into interproximal regions, where fluoride is most effective in the prevention of caries.

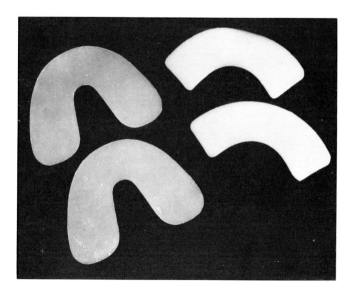

Figure 35. *A sample of wax application trays. The pair on the right are waxy in consistency while the pair on the left are formed from a smooth thermoplastic material.*

Preventive Dentistry

When the application tray is removed from the mouth after the four-minute exposure, the reverse series of events should occur. The agent in interproximal regions reverts to its gel state on removal of pressure from the tray, and a thin layer should remain in situ after the tray is removed.

Fluoride Application Trays or Mouthpieces

In my opinion, the most important aspect in the use of fluoride gels for topical application is the design of the application trays that are used clinically. Because the APF gels are viscous, poorly fitting trays may result in contact only between gel and freely exposed enamel surfaces, and not with interproximal regions. Even when using the new thixotropic gel it is essential to use a well-fitting application tray. Because the design of fluoride trays is important and many different types are available, it is worth examining a selection.

Wax Trays

Probably the earliest available application trays for use with APF gels were wax trays (Figure 35). Several types are available. These range from rather sticky and waxy agents to smooth thermoplastic materials. The former types are to be avoided because they tend to leave a waxy coating on the enamel surface which will reduce contact of the fluoride agent with the tooth surface. The trays are usually available in one size only, and are trimmed if necessary at the chairside. They are then moulded into an arch, upper and lower trays being identical. The trays are then tried in the mouth, modified, readapted if necessary and air-dried. Fluoride gel is then poured into the tray.

In my opinion most operators overfill application trays with fluoride gel. This tends to extrude from the tray and runs into the posterior of the oral cavity. A single strip of gel should be poured into the tray from the nozzle of the polythene container, beginning at one extremity of the tray and passing slowly to the other. The wax trays are inserted over the previously cleaned and dried teeth, a saliva ejector placed between them (Figure 36), and the patient

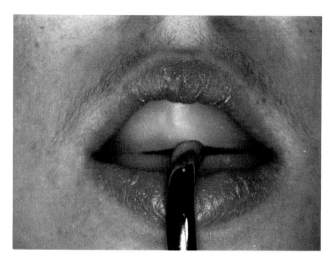

Figure 36. *Wax fluoride application trays in situ with a saliva ejector between them.*

instructed to close his mouth gently. The operator should then try to shape the wax trays to the buccal contours of the teeth using gentle but firm finger pressure.

If the patient is old enough, he should be asked to attempt the same procedure on the lingual and palatal aspects using the tip of his tongue. This way fluoride gel may be taken further into interproximal sites. After a four-minute exposure, the trays are removed, excess gel wiped away from the teeth with gauze, and the patient told not to rinse out his mouth for about 30 minutes.

Advantages. Both arches are treated at the one time.

Disadvantages. The time taken to trim trays; cost, because trays are disposable; and doubts about the efficacy of fluoride application to interproximal sites.

Polyvinyl Application Trays

There are a number of polyvinyl fluoride application trays available conforming to the general design as shown in Figure 37. Their

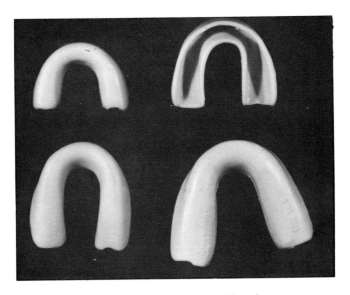

Figure 37. *A sample of polyvinyl application trays.*

main disadvantages are:

1. The distal aspects of the trays are open-ended and hence flouride gel tends to run out of the trays into the posterior of the oral cavity causing the patient to gag.

2. The trays are wide in their lateral dimensions resulting in very little pressure being applied to the gel. Pressure is required to aid its flow into interproximal regions.

Thus the main contact is between freely exposed enamel surfaces (occlusal, buccal and lingual) and gel, with little material penetrating into the interproximal regions. With some polyvinyl trays, filter paper liners are supplied (Figure 38) so that the trays can be used in conjunction with fluoride solutions. In the author's opinion this is of little merit because, at best, only the cusps, cuspal slopes and buccal and lingual surfaces could possibly come into contact with the fluoride-moistened filter paper inserts. It is unfortunate that so many poor features are incorporated in the design of such trays because they are well accepted by patients (Figure 39).

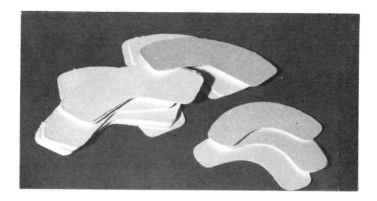

Figure 38. *Filter paper liners for use with polyvinyl trays when a fluoride solution is used for topical application.*

Advantages. Both arches are treated at the one time and the trays are simple and quick to use. Cost is low because trays are reusable after cold sterilization.

Disadvantages. Trays are open-ended and gel flows out causing the patient to gag. They are also too wide laterally, resulting in no pressure to force the gel interproximally.

Impression Materials

An alginate impression may be taken of the arch and used as a special tray for the application of a fluoride gel. However, there is no need to use an upper impression tray to treat the maxillary arch because the use of a lower tray will leave the palate free.

After taking the impression the fitting surface of the alginate is air-dried and a small amount of fluoride gel poured into the relevant indentations. The tray is then reinserted over the cleaned and dried teeth. In this manner fluoride gel is probably forced into the interproximal sites by the well-fitting impression material. There have been fears that calcium ions from the alginate will react with fluoride ions from the gel and 'inactivate' the system. Since only the monolayer in contact with the enamel surface is vital in the transport of fluoride ions into the enamel surface, the above

73

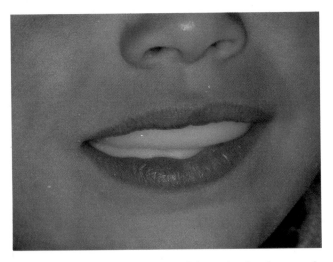

Figure 39. *A six-year-old child with polyvinyl trays in place.*

reaction is unlikely to affect the system adversely, because only fluoride ions on the outer aspect of the gel, i.e. in contact with the tray, might be affected. Other impression materials, such as silicone rubber, rubber base, etc., may also be used this way. However, these materials are relatively expensive.

Advantages. This is a simple technique using materials always available in the dental office.

Disadvantages. Each arch is treated separately, the cost of impression tray and material for each application is high and it takes time to make the impression before application of fluoride gel.

Vacuum-Moulded 'Fluoride Splints'

Vacuum-moulded splints may be constructed for the patient in the same manner as splints used for immobilization of anterior mobile teeth after trauma. The splints are vacuum moulded over plaster models of the upper and lower arches (Figure 40). The splints are trimmed so that the peripheral regions are almost level with the gingival margins (Figure 41). After cleaning and drying the teeth, a

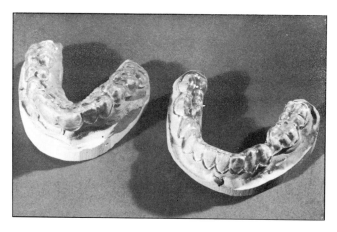

Figure 40. *Plaster models on which vacuum-moulded 'fluoride splints' are constructed.*

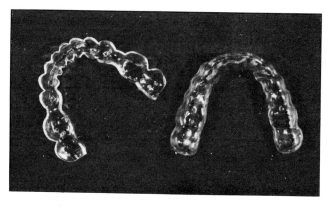

Figure 41. *A pair of vacuum-moulded fluoride splints similar in design and construction to splints made for the immobilization of mobile incisors after trauma.*

small amount of fluoride gel is poured into each fluoride splint. When in place, fluoride gel is accurately spread over relevant tooth surfaces and good interproximal flow should result (Figure 42). The splints need to be remade when the dentition is modified, which occurs relatively often during the mixed dentition period.

75

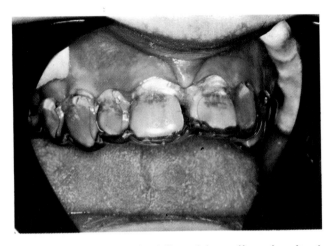

Figure 42. *Vacuum-moulded fluoride splints in situ in a patient with dysplastic enamel.*

Advantages. Both arches are treated at the same time and the fit is accurate with good interproximal flow. The splints are comfortable for the patient because there is no bulk.

Disadvantages. Laboratory costs for construction are high and the splints have to be remade when the dentition is modified.

Combined Polyvinyl Applicator Tray and Disposable Foam Insert

The Flura-Tray System (Kerr, Sybron Corp.) combines the use of a flexible polyvinyl application tray with a disposable foam insert (Figure 43). The tray system consists of two trays hinged together so that both arches are treated at the same time. Just before use, a foam insert is tucked into the relevant size of tray (Figure 44) and fluoride gel poured around the dual system. The trays are folded so that their 'backs' or outer surfaces are in contact, and inserted over both arches which have been previously cleaned and dried. The patient is then instructed to simulate a mild chewing action during the four-minute exposure. The disposable foam insert is constructed from a hydrophilic material which swells on absorbing

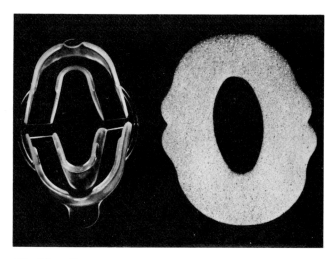

Figure 43. *The Flura-Tray System (Kerr Sybron Corp.) in which a pair of hinged polyvinyl trays are used in combination with a disposable foam insert.*

fluid. In this manner, the insert adapts itself close to the buccal and lingual aspects of the teeth, ensuring good contact between fluoride gel and enamel surfaces. It is hoped that the chewing action will carry the fluoride gel into interproximal sites. The double-tray system is well tolerated by children (Figure 45), although pressure in the sulcus from the thickened polythene rim of the tray sometimes causes some mild discomfort.

Advantages. Both arches are treated at the same time, the foam insert keeps the gel in contact with the teeth and the cost is low because trays are reused.

Disadvantages. The initial cost of the system is high and the foam inserts are disposable, although low in cost. Some discomfort to the patient may also result from the thickened rim of the tray.

Air-Cushion Fluoride Trays

These trays (Ion Brand, 3M Company) consist essentially of an air-filled rubber membrane which is contained in a plastic tray

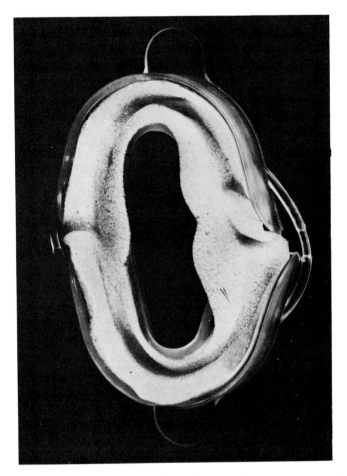

Figure 44. *Just before use the disposable foam insert is tucked into the tray and fluoride gel poured over it. The trays are then folded back on themselves and inserted into the mouth so that both arches are treated at the same time.*

(Figures 46 and 47). Before use an absorbent, disposable paper insert is placed in the rubber membrane, and fluoride gel poured into the tray in the usual manner. A plastic cheek retractor is supplied with the kit. This is used to isolate the entire arch from the

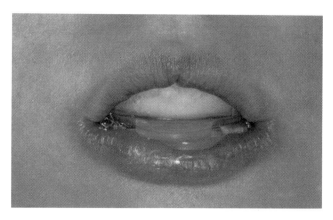

Figure 45. *Patient with Flura-Tray (Kerr) application trays in place. Both arches are treated at the same time; the foam insert only is disposable.*

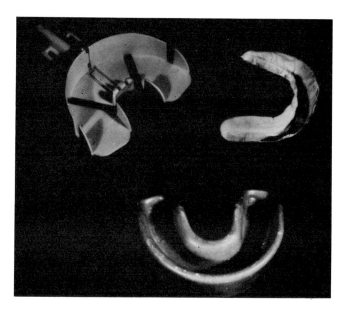

Figure 46. *An exploded view of an Air-Cushion Fluoride Tray (Ion Brand, 3M Company) consisting of an air-filled rubber membrane, a paper insert and a plastic supporting tray.*

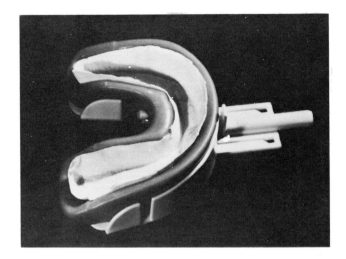

Figure 47. *The Air-Cushion Fluoride Tray assembled for use. Fluoride gel is poured into the paper insert.*

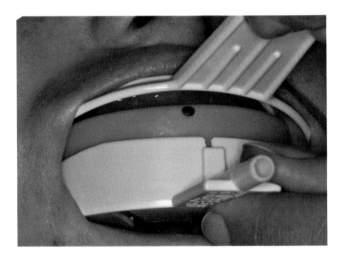

Figure 48. *An Air-Cushion Fluoride Tray (Ion Brand, 3M) being inserted over an upper arch. A plastic cheek retractor, supplied with kit, is used to isolate the entire arch from the cheeks to allow drying of the teeth before insertion of the tray. Once the tray is in position the cheek retractor is removed.*

cheeks to allow drying of teeth before insertion of the tray (Figure 48). When the tray is inserted, air in the rubber membrane is compressed causing the tray to conform to the contours of the teeth. The rubber membrane helps to seal out saliva while holding the fluoride-saturated paper insert in close contact with enamel surfaces. This system certainly aids the flow of fluoride gel into interproximal sites.

The tray is removed after a four-minute exposure, leaving the paper insert still in close contact with the teeth. In this way it is possible to see how the liner has been adapted to the teeth. The liner is removed and excess gel wiped off with gauze. As with other topical fluoride treatments, the patient is told not to rinse or drink for about 30 minutes. The trays are relatively large. The author finds that it is only possible to treat one arch at a time (Figure 48). Although this may be a disadvantage, the air-filled membrane is extremely comfortable and is well accepted by young children.

Advantages. This tray is very comfortable for the patient, and close contact between fluoride gel and enamel surfaces is maintained.

Disadvantages. Each arch is treated separately and the initial cost of the system is high.

Disposable Trays

AlphaTrays (Amalgamated Dental Co., London) are purpose-designed disposable foam–plastic trays, colour coded in three sizes (Figure 49). The trough has sufficient depth to allow full coverage of the anterior teeth. It widens towards the posterior of the tray to allow for posterior teeth. This design gives maximum coverage of teeth in either arch and, by conforming with the contours of the dental arch, considerably reduces the amount of gel required for each application.

The posterior dam prevents gel from escaping and causing discomfort to the patient. Because of the close fit of the trays, gel seldom escapes and a saliva ejector is not essential. In addition, the gel is pressed close to the enamel surfaces because of the relatively narrow trough which expands when the teeth are forced in. In this

81

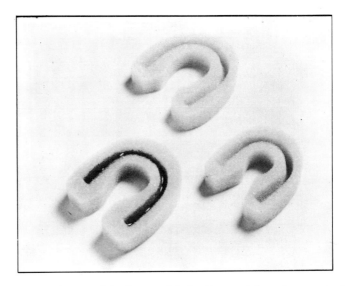

Figure 49. *Disposable foam AlphaTrays (Amalgamated Dental, London). These are made in three sizes and are colour coded. The posterior dam prevents gel from escaping and causing discomfort to the patient. Gel seldom leaks from any part of the tray because of its close fit, a feature which aids in the flow of gel into the interproximal regions.*

way fluoride gel is pressed into interproximal sites. Excess saliva is taken up by the sponge-like foam without interfering with the mechanism of fluoride uptake by the enamel. These trays are a little more difficult to use at first, compared with the polyvinyl type, because they are flexible.

The upper tray is inserted first and held in place with the left hand by placing the index finger over the upper right quadrant, and the middle finger over the left quadrant. The lower tray is then 'puddled' into place, and the patient told to close his mouth gently. If a saliva ejector is to be used, this is placed between the trays (Figure 50). After a short while these trays are as easy to use as non-flexible trays, but have the advantages of good contact of gel with free and interproximal enamel, coupled with extreme comfort. After a four-minute exposure, the trays are removed and

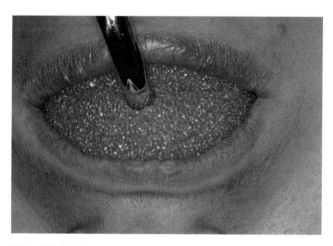

Figure 50. *AlphaTrays (Amalgamated Dental) in position with a saliva ejector between them. The pink trays are the smallest of the three colour-coded sizes.*

disposed of, and excess gel wiped off the teeth.

The Pacemaker Corp. (Portland, Oregon) have recently introduced a preformed disposable fluoride tray, 'Centrays', made from a soft flexible material and available in three sizes (Figure 51). Separate moulds are used for maxillary and mandibular arches. Upper trays are white in colour whereas lower trays are blue. These trays are extremely well accepted by young patients and both arches can be treated at the same time.

Advantages. Both arches are treated at the one time and the trays are extremely comfortable. Close contact between enamel and gel is maintained.

Disadvantages. The trays are disposable but low in cost, initially and at replacement.

Prophylaxis

It is well accepted that teeth must be cleaned thoroughly before applying fluorides topically. However, no scientifically based

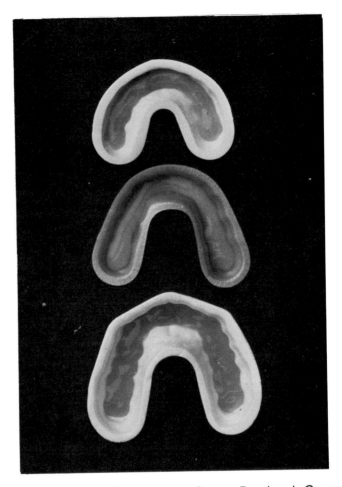

Figure 51. *Centrays (Pacemaker Corp., Portland, Oregon) are made in three sizes and colour-coded for upper and lower moulds. These are extremely comfortable for patients and are highly efficient.*

studies have shown unequivocally that prophylaxis before the topical application of fluorides is of significant benefit. Although such trials are in progress, it is reasonable to continue with the prophylaxis regimen before the clinical application of fluorides. Since

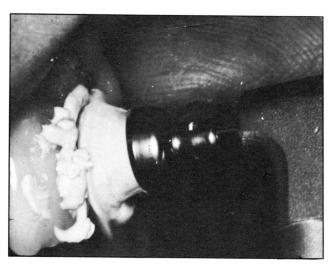

Figure 52. *The prophylaxis: a rotating rubber cup cleaning the buccal aspect of a tooth with prophylaxis paste.*

interproximal surfaces benefit significantly from topically applied fluorides, these sites should also be cleaned thoroughly. To do this efficiently dental floss must be used. Unwaxed floss should be used because the waxed type will leave an impervious waxy coating on the enamel surface which, in turn, will adversely affect penetration of fluoride ions into enamel. A rubber cup should be used for prophylaxis (Figure 52). The author finds that the 'Youngs' type of rubber cup is highly suitable because on rotation, the flexible periphery tends to splay out on contact with the enamel surface. This way it is possible to penetrate and clean, to some extent, into interproximal regions.

Because prophylaxis paste is used with a rubber cup, it is reasonable to select a fluoride-containing paste, although its use on enamel alone should not necessarily be regarded as an efficient topical fluoride treatment. There are several fluoride-containing prophylaxis pastes available containing either sodium fluoride, stannous fluoride or APF. Individual sachets of APF prophylaxis paste are also available.

Home Fluoride Treatment

For children or adults with problems of severe or rampant caries, an intensive course of fluoride application may be prescribed for home use. The daily home use of a fluoride gel containing 0.6 per cent fluoride ion has been recommended (Wei 1976). A number of commercially available APF gels are now available for home use (Pacemaker Corp., Lorvic Corp. and Hoyt Co.). The use of suitable trays is recommended in the application of fluoride gels as part of the home fluoride treatment. A prescription for 250 ml of 0.6 per cent fluoride ion APF gel should last approximately three months. Home fluoride treatment should be commenced prior to and during restorative treatment. Once control of the active phase of caries has been achieved, therapy should be continued with lower potency fluoride supplements such as fluoride mouthrinses. Home fluoride treatment is contraindicated in young children who may swallow a significant portion of the fluoride agent. This could lead to the possibility of enamel fluorosis.

Suggested Topical Fluoride Regimen

1. Carry out a rubber cup prophylaxis using prophylaxis paste containing fluoride. Use unwaxed floss interproximally.

2. Wash and dry enamel surfaces.

3. Materials for topical application. Use new thixotropic gel (Gel II or AlphaGel) with comfortable trays, either Centrays or air-cushion trays. Select correct size trays, and insert appropriate amount of fluoride gel.

4. Dry teeth in upper arch and insert tray. If using air-cushion trays, leave upper tray in situ for four minutes, and then repeat procedure with the lower tray. If using Centrays, both arches are treated simultaneously. A clock with a large dial and a large sweep second hand should be used to time the four-minute exposure. The child can hold the clock, giving him something to do.

5. After the four-minute exposure, remove trays and wipe off excess gel from teeth with gauze. The patient should not rinse out his mouth for about 30 minutes. Topical application of fluorides

should be carried out during the school vacation. This way children can have three topical applications of fluoride each year.

Dangers

The acute lethal dose of fluoride is about 50 mg per kilogram of bodyweight (Cox and Hodge 1950). However, as little as 3 mg per kilogram of bodyweight is apparently sufficient to produce early symptoms of acute fluoride poisoning (the average five-year-old child weighs about 20 kg). Should a child swallow a fluoride solution it is likely that vomiting will occur. The antidote to fluoride poisoning was discussed in Chapter 2. From the toxicity point of view it is worth remembering that, for equal volumes, stannous fluoride solution contains twice as much fluoride as an APF solution. In addition, the tin in SnF_2 could further contribute to the toxicity problem if an aliquot was swallowed.

References

Braden, M., *J. Dent. Res.*, 1974, **53**, 1089 (Abst).

Brudevold, F., Savory, A., Gardner, D. E., Spinelli, M. and Speirs, R., *Arch. Oral Biol.*, 1963, **8**, 167.

Clarkson, B. H. and Silverstone, L. M., *J. Int. Assoc. Dent. Child.*, 1974, **5**, 27.

Cox, G. J. and Hodge, H. C., *J. Am. Dent. Assoc.*, 1950, **40**, 440.

Muhler, J. C., *J. Periodont.*, 1957, **28**, 281.

Swieterman, R. P., Muhler, J. C. and Swenson, H. M., *J. Periodont.*, 1961, **32**, 131.

Wei, S. H. Y., *Fluorides: An Update for Dental Practice*, S. Moss and S. H. Y. Wei (Eds), Medcom, New York, 1976.

6. Topical Fluorides: Mouth Rinses, Dentifrices, Pastes and Varnishes

Fluoride Mouth Rinses

Fluoride mouth rinsing is one of several topical fluoride techniques available which may be particularly suited to community dental health programmes. The results of early trials were disappointing (Bibby et al. 1946). It was not until a decade ago that renewed interest was shown by workers in Sweden. In one study (Torell and Siberg 1962), the use of monthly 0.2 per cent sodium or potassium fluoride rinses demonstrated substantial reductions in anterior approximal caries. Later it was found that the addition of manganese ions enhanced the effect of potassium fluoride (Gerdin and Torell 1969).

In a comprehensive multigroup trial (Torell and Ericsson 1965), the unsupervised daily use of an 0.05 per cent sodium fluoride mouth rinse over a two-year period was shown to reduce the incidence of caries by about 50 per cent in 10- to 12-year-old children. This reduction was significantly greater than that obtained by supervised rinsing every second week with an 0.2 per cent sodium fluoride solution in the same trial. In this latter group, only a 21 per cent caries reduction was found, indicating the importance of frequent exposure in the use of topical fluorides. A 44 per cent reduction in DMF increment was produced in a 20-month trial in the USA (Horowitz et al. 1971) with weekly rinsing with a solution of 0.2 per cent sodium fluoride.

In a further multigroup trial Koch (1967) determined the effect of fluoride toothpastes and fluoride mouth rinses on caries incidence in Swedish schoolchildren. Two sodium fluoride solutions were used, 0.5 per cent and 0.05 per cent. Ten millilitres of the 0.5

per cent solution was used for each rinse, containing about 23 mg of fluoride. The 0.5 per cent rinse was prepared by dissolving 10 ml of 0.6 per cent NaF in 100 ml of tap water. This solution contained 27 mg of fluoride. Three study groups were used to test the fluoride rinses. There was a 23 per cent reduction in DMFS scored in the fluoride group compared with the control. When the caries increments were considered for various tooth surfaces it was found that occlusal caries was not affected by the fluoride rinse.

The largest reduction in caries was on buccal and approximal surfaces. The children who rinsed only when they attended the school clinic used the mouthwash three to four times a year on average. The third group used a 0.05 per cent NaF solution. However, they used 110 ml of this solution and had to use all of this volume. Therefore, the total fluoride content was slightly higher for this group than for the other two groups. The children rinsed about three times a year. Using a 0.05 per cent solution three times a year, no reduction in caries was obtained. It was concluded that daily rinsing with such a weak solution would probably be necessary before a reduction in caries was obtained.

Two years after the above trial had ended, Koch (1969) re-examined the children who had taken part in the rinsing once every two weeks with 0.5 per cent NaF. One hundred and forty children were available for re-examination. A difference was found between control and test groups but this difference was not statistically significant. Thus, no prolonged caries preventive effect could be found two years after the end of a programme based on rinsing once every two weeks with 0.5 per cent sodium fluoride solution. It appears that the beneficial effect of supervised mouth rinsing with fluoride solution can only be maintained if mouth rinsing is continued. Koch's study on mouth rinsing is one of the largest so far reported and is the only one in which the caries increment was determined after the fluoride rinsing programme had ended.

Sodium Fluoride

In a recent study carried out in the UK (Rugg-Gunn et al. 1973) more than 400 15-year-old subjects completed a three-year double-blind trial testing the daily supervised use of a mouth rinse containing 0.05 per cent sodium fluoride. The control rinse was similar except for the omission of fluoride. There was a 36 per cent reduction (3.7 DMFS) over the three-year period. The highest percentage reductions were found on anterior approximal and free smooth surfaces. No adverse effects on oral soft tissues were found, and ingestion of fluoride from the rinses was low. With respect to cost-effectiveness, it was considered that one supervisor could organize a daily mouth-rinsing programme for 800 subjects at a cost of about $8.00 (£4) per child per year. These results were in agreement with other fluoride mouth-rinsing studies (Koch 1967) in that caries reductions were greatest on free smooth surfaces and anterior approximal surfaces.

Although it had previously been suggested that rinsing with an 0.5 per cent sodium fluoride solution every two weeks had an unfavourable effect upon gingival health (Koch and Lindhe 1967), this was not observed in the British trial (Rugg-Gunn et al. 1973). This lack of adverse effect on gingival health has also been demonstrated in other studies. A further double-blind British study carried out over two years (Brandt et al. 1972), with supervised 0.2 per cent sodium fluoride rinsing for one minute, produced its greatest caries reduction on posterior approximal surfaces. With respect to the posterior teeth only, a 48 per cent reduction was found. This study therefore differs from others with respect to the surfaces showing the greatest reductions.

Acidulated Phosphate Fluoride

In addition to sodium fluoride, acidulated phosphate fluoride (APF) has also been used in mouth rinse studies. One such study compared three groups of 8- to 11-year-old children over a three-year period (Aasenden et al. 1972). One group received daily 5 ml sodium fluoride rinses containing 0.02 per cent fluoride, whereas the second group used an acidulated phosphate fluoride rinse, also containing the equivalent of 0.02 per cent fluoride. The third group received a neutral placebo. The solutions were kept in the mouth for one minute and then swallowed. At the end of the study, reductions in DMFS of 27 per cent and 30 per cent were found in the neutral sodium fluoride and APF groups, respectively. Enamel biopsies showed that the APF solution was superior to sodium fluoride in depositing fluoride in intact enamel.

Effectiveness and Acceptability of Rinses

Heifetz et al. (1973) also investigated the effectiveness of neutral sodium fluoride and acidulated phosphate fluoride incorporated into mouth rinses used on a weekly basis. Nine hundred and forty-seven children, 10 to 12 years of age, were included in the trial and the fluoride concentration used (0.3 per cent) was the highest reported to date. Of three randomly selected groups, the first rinsed weekly at school (24 times per year) with an artificially sweetened neutral 0.6 per cent solution of sodium fluoride (0.3 per cent F). The second group used an acidulated phosphate fluoride solution at pH 4 which also had a 0.3 per cent fluoride concentration. The third group rinsed weekly with a placebo solution.

This study terminated in the second year because the taste of the acidulated phosphate fluoride (APF) solution was not acceptable to the children. Similar results were found in the groups rinsing with either the NaF or the APF solutions. These groups had 23 per cent and 20 per cent fewer new carious surfaces, respectively. The addition of radiographic findings to the clinical data resulted in final reductions of 38 per cent and 27 per cent, respectively.

All rinsing studies referred to so far have been carried out in non-fluoride areas. Radike et al. (1973) evaluated the effect of rinsing in a 20-month study using a rinse containing 0.1 per cent stannous fluoride. This was conducted on 900 children, 8 to 13 years of age, who resided in an area where the water had been fluoridated to a level of 1 ppm. The children rinsed three times, for 10, 20 and 30 seconds, every other school day. The children in study and control groups had a similar caries experience at the start of the study. Of the two dental examiners employed, both found a small reduction in caries increment at the end of the trial. This is an interesting result, because some benefit was apparently obtained by rinsing in addition to that derived from the consumption of fluoridated drinking water.

Thus, many studies have shown that fluoride incorporated into a mouth rinse is effective in reducing the incidence of dental caries over a period of one to three years. This has been observed in fluoride and non-fluoride areas. However, the observation by Koch (1969) is important in that no difference between study and control groups was observed two years after cessation of mouth rinsing. It appears, therefore, that the beneficial effect of mouth rinsing with fluoride solutions can only be maintained if continued. Further studies are necessary to investigate whether benefits are maintained if the rinsing regimen is gradually phased down to, for example, monthly rinses. Alternatively, it may be sufficient to change to another fluoride regimen, such as annual topically applied fluorides, to maintain the benefits gained by fluoride rinsing.

This summary demonstrates that fluoride mouth rinsing may provide an answer to the problems of insufficient professional manpower and excessive costs that currently hinder topical fluoride programmes.

Fluoride Dentifrices

Since a large segment of the population uses a dentifrice in conjunction with toothbrushing, the incorporation of fluoride into dentifrices is a logical and practical approach to the problem of delivering topical fluorides to a large number of people. Many studies on fluoride-containing dentifrices have been carried out. It can be concluded that several formulations containing stannous fluoride, sodium fluoride or sodium monofluorophosphate have anticariogenic properties, and reduce caries by 15 to 30 per cent. However, because of the inability of young children to expectorate efficiently, fluoride-containing dentifrices should not be used until a child is four years of age.

The abrasives and other ingredients of dentifrices must be compatible with the dentifrice's fluoride system. Abrasives such as calcium pyrophosphate, insoluble sodium metaphosphate and acrylic particles have shown compatibility with their respective fluorides and have been reviewed in detail elsewhere (Duckworth 1968; Heifetz and Horowitz 1972). Dentifrices are readily available proprietary products and, therefore, the levels of fluoride have to be kept low—in the region of 0.1 per cent—to avoid the danger of ingestion of possibly toxic quantities by children.

Hargreaves and Chester (1973) conducted trials in which they investigated the effect of increasing the concentration of mono-fluorophosphate (MFP) to two per cent. The caries reductions found over a three-year period did not differ markedly from those in studies using lower concentrations of MFP. The greatest effect was found on smooth surfaces. One year after termination of the study 221 children were re-examined. It was reported (Hargreaves et al. 1975) that a statistically significant difference in DMF increment between test and placebo groups still remained.

Although the caries reduction produced by using fluoride-containing dentifrices is low, an average of 20 per cent reduction in DMFS, it is nevertheless significant. Because this technique does not depend upon professional or supervised care, it represents a very useful and important part of a caries preventive programme.

Fluoride-Containing Prophylaxis Pastes

Early in the development of topical fluoride programmes, it was recommended that before application of the fluoride agent, teeth should be cleaned with a polishing paste. A rubber-cup prophylaxis has therefore been an integral part of the topical fluoride therapy. It would be an attractive proposition if, by incorporating a fluoride compound into a polishing paste, prophylaxis and topical fluoride application could be carried out in one procedure. However, because the fluoride ion is highly reactive, it readily forms complexes with the other constituents of the polishing paste and therefore tends to become inactivated.

The collective findings with an eight to nine per cent stannous fluoride–lava pumice prophylaxis paste indicate that its use alone on a semiannual basis will produce a modest caries preventive effect. The cariostatic effect, however, is not comparable to that produced by topical application of fluoride preceded by prophylaxis with a non-fluoride paste. Thus, the recommendation for using a fluoride-containing prophylaxis paste is a controversial subject. The more recent development of zirconium silicate–stannous fluoride and silicone dioxide–acidulated phosphate fluoride prophylaxis pastes may produce more successful results. No clinical trials have been reported which confirm the promising results obtained in the laboratory with fluoride-containing polishing pastes.

Prophylaxis with a fluoride-containing polishing paste should not replace the topical application of fluorides. At present there is inadequate data to recommend any professionally applied fluoride-polishing paste as the sole fluoride agent in a topical fluoride programme. A thorough prophylaxis will remove a thin, but significant, layer of surface enamel of the order of 2 to 4 μm (Vrbic et al. 1967). This layer is rich in fluoride and highly mineralized. Therefore, if prophylaxis is not to be followed by topical application of a concentrated fluoride solution or gel, a fluoride-containing polishing paste should be used initially for cleaning the teeth to replace the fluoride which is removed.

Prophylaxis conventionally precedes a professionally applied topical fluoride treatment to make enamel surfaces readily accessible to the fluoride agent. The absence of prophylaxis preceding the topical application has been shown to reduce benefits (Gron and Brudevold 1967). However, a study by Tinanoff et al. (1974) showed that provided plaque was removed by thorough brushing and flossing, the necessity for a prophylaxis before a topical fluoride application was questionable. Although it is not clear whether a fluoride-containing prophylaxis paste enhances the effect of the topical application, there are no contraindications to using one in conjunction with a subsequent topical fluoride application.

Fluoride Varnishes

In recent years varnishes containing fluoride have been produced in an attempt to maintain the fluoride ion in intimate contact with the enamel surface for longer periods than conventional topical fluoride applications. After initial studies on extracted teeth, favourable results have been obtained in clinical trials. In one study (Heuser and Schmidt 1968), a 30 per cent reduction in caries increment between the study and control groups was found over a 15-month period. The varnish yielded 2.26 per cent available fluoride and was stated to be remarkably water tolerant so that it could cover moist teeth.

In a recent in vitro study (Koch and Petersson 1972) a high concentration of fluoride was found in the outermost layer of enamel after treatment with the varnish. In a recent clinical trial 376 five-year-old children were treated with a fluoride varnish using a half-month technique (Murray et al. 1977). At the end of the second year, only 20 per cent of the control first permanent molars were carious compared with 13 per cent of the test first permanent molars. Further long-term clinical studies should be carried out before this method can be recommended as an effective caries preventive agent. At present fluoride varnishes should be regarded as experimental agents.

References

Aasenden, R., de Paola, P. F. and Brudevold, F., *Arch. Oral. Biol.*, 1972, **17**, 1705.

Bibby, B. G., Zander, H. A., McKelleget, M. and Labunsky, B., *J. Dent. Res.*, 1946, **25**, 207.

Brandt, R. S., Slack, G. L. and Waller, D., *Proc. Br. Paediatr. Soc.*, 1972, **2**, 464.

Duckworth, R., *Br. Dent. J.*, 1968, **124**, 505.

Gerdin, P. O. and Torell, P., *Caries Res.*, 1969, **3**, 99.

Gron, P. and Brudevold, F., *J. Dent. Child.*, 1967, **34**, 123.

Hargreaves, J. A. and Chester, C. G., *Comm. Dent. Oral Epidem.*, 1973, **1**, 41.

Hargreaves, J. A., Chester, C. G. and Wagg, B. J., *Caries Res.*, 1975, **9**, 291.

Heifetz, S. B. and Horowitz, H. S., *Fluorides and Dental Caries*, Newbrun, E. (Ed.), p. 22, Charles C. Thomas, Springfield, Massachusetts, USA, 1972.

Heifetz, S. B., Driscoll, W. S. and Creighton, W. E., *J. Am. Dent. Assoc.*, 1973, **87**, 364.

Heuser, H. and Schmidt, H. F. M., *Stoma*, 1968, **2**, 91.

Horowitz, H. S., Creighton, W. E. and McClendon, B. J., *Arch. Oral Biol.*, 1971, **16**, 609.

Koch, G., *Odont. Revy*, 1967, **18**, (Suppl. vol), 12.

Koch, G. L., *Odont. Revy*, 1969, **20**, 323.

Koch, G. and Lindhe, J., *J. Periodont. Res.*, 1967, **2**, 533.

Koch, G. and Petersson, L. G., *Odont. Revy*, 1972, **23**, 437.

Murray, J. J., Winter, G. B. and Hurst, C. P., *Br. Dent. J.*, 1977, **143**, 11.

Preventive Dentistry

Radike, A. W., Gish, C. W., Paterson, J. K. and Segreto, V. A., *J. Am. Dent. Assoc.*, 1973, **86**, 404.

Rugg-Gunn, A. J., Holloway, P. J. and Davies, T. G. H., *Br. Dent. J.*, 1973, **135**, 353.

Tinanoff, N., Wei, S. H. Y. and Parkins, F. M., *J. Am. Dent. Assoc.*, 1974, **88**, 384.

Torell, P. and Ericsson, Y., *Acta Odont. Scand.*, 1965, **23**, 287.

Torell, P. and Siberg, A., *Odont. Revy*, 1962, **13**, 62.

Vrbic, V., Brudevold, F. and McCann, H. G., *Helv. Odont. Acta*, 1967, **11**, 21.

7. Fissure Sealants

Numerous studies show that fluoridation of public water supplies and the use of fluoride preparations reduce caries significantly. While the approximal sites show the greatest reductions, the occlusal surfaces of posterior teeth benefit the least (Backer Dirks et al. 1961).

A number of techniques have been proposed in an attempt to prevent occlusal caries. Hyatt (1923) suggested the technique of prophylactic odontotomy whereby occlusal fissures were filled, but this was not widely accepted because it was necessary to prepare cavities in sound teeth. The use of chemical agents to seal pits and fissures, such as ammoniacal silver nitrate (Klein and Knutson 1942), zinc chloride and potassium ferrocyanide (Ast et al. 1950) met with little success, as did the use of copper cement (Miller 1950). The development of new synthetic resins led to the possibility of sealing occlusal fissures with adhesive materials requiring no cavity preparation.

Early work with the epoxy resins was unsuccessful because the bond strength of these adhesives to the enamel surface was poor, due to the presence of water in the tissue. The introduction of the cyanoacrylate group of adhesives seemed likely to overcome this difficulty by using a small amount of water for polymerization. Initial application was found in medicine for the non-suture closure of arterial incisions (Nathan et al. 1960). However, methyl-2-cyanoacrylate was found to be unsatisfactory because it was degraded in the tissues with some histotoxicity as a result of degradation byproducts of formaldehyde and methyl cyanoacetate (Cameron et al. 1965).

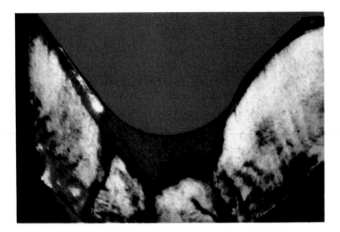

Figure 53. *Longitudinal ground section through a tooth showing the presence of a fissure sealant in the occlusal fissure. Stagnation areas present in the fissure have been eliminated by the sealant which has a smooth surface contour. The section is examined in quinoline with the polarizing microscope.*

Clinical Trials

In a developed community dependent upon an average diet, the high prevalence of dental caries cannot be controlled by reparative techniques alone. Caries prevention programmes must be run in addition to restorative procedures if the disease is to be controlled. From all available evidence, fissure sealants are likely to play an important role in caries prevention by augmenting fluoride and other techniques, because they are intended to protect caries-susceptible surfaces that are least benefited by fluoride. Because caries of the occlusal surface accounts for approximately half the caries in English children during their time at school (Oswald 1973), and because it is the surface least protected by fluoride, the use of fissure sealants on occlusal surfaces can have a highly significant caries preventive effect (Figure 53).

Methyl-2-cyanoacrylate

A number of sealant trials have been carried out to date and others are in progress. Although initial trials with methyl-2-cyanoacrylate produced significant results (Cueto and Buonocore 1967), reapplication every six months was found to be necessary. A trial using this material in Britain (Parkhouse and Winter 1971) showed an almost total failure by the six-month recall period. Although these workers used slightly different parameters in their use of the material, it displayed failure in the hands of others. Crabb and Wilson (1971) showed that the bond strength of methyl-2-cyanocrylate was reduced to one-sixth of its dry value by immersion in water for 24 hours. This factor may have been significant regarding retention of the material. As far as the author is aware, there is no fissure sealant available commercially which is based entirely on the methyl-2-cyanoacrylate formulation.

Bis-GMA

The next stage in the development of the technique was the use of a new material as a fissure sealant, based on bisphenol A-glycidyl methacrylate (Bis-GMA). This material was developed by Bowen (1962) at the National Bureau of Standards, Washington, DC. A pilot study carried out by Roydhouse (1968) showed the potential of the material as a sealant.

Nuva-Seal

Buonocore and his colleagues then modified this Bis-GMA sealant system by using a UV light-sensitive catalyst, benzoin methyl ether. The material (Nuva-Seal, Caulk Co., Milford, Delaware) was polymerized by longwave UV light using the Spectroline lamp.

The Rochester Trial

Two-year results of a clinical trial using this system, carried out in Rochester, NY, were reported by Buonocore (1971). He found that a single application of the sealant was almost completely effective in protecting occlusal surfaces from caries. Occlusal caries was reported in only one out of 113 treated surfaces. However, in his trial, teeth were selected on the basis of having well-defined pits and fissures. In later trials carried out by other workers, criteria for selection of teeth, such as specific morphological features, were not used. This may be one reason why the results of other trials are less striking.

The Kalispell Trial

More recently Horowitz et al. (1974) reported on the effectiveness of Nuva-Seal in a two-year trial in Kalispell, Montana. The children who took part in the trial were of two age groups—five- to eight-year-olds and 10- to 14-year-olds. The sealant was applied using portable equipment in a school environment. After one year of the trial (Table 3), results on 900 pairs of homologous teeth showed an 81 per cent reduction in caries and an 88 per cent total retention of sealant (McCune et al. 1973). After the second year of the trial (Table 3), the sealant was reported as showing a 67 per cent reduction in caries relative to controls. Seventy-three per cent of test teeth showed full retention of the sealant. Failure of the sealant was recorded if the treated tooth was either carious, restored or extracted. If a two-surface (Class II) restoration was found in the tooth, although it may have been inserted as a result of approximal caries, it was counted as a sealant failure in this trial.

Restorative treatment of approximal caries was more relevant than in the Rochester trial, because Rochester is optimally fluoridated. Thus, sealant failures estimated in the Kalispell study as a result of approximal caries would have been much higher than those in the fluoridated region. The results, however, are good regarding caries reduction, especially when it is remembered that the sealant was placed in less than optimal surroundings, using portable equipment.

Horowitz and co-workers reported their four-year results in 1975. After four years, 50 per cent of all sites showed complete retention of sealant, with 16 per cent showing partial retention. For all sites remaining fully sealed there was a 99 per cent reduction in caries. For sites showing partial retention of material a 90 per cent reduction in caries was recorded. In addition, there was a six per cent reduction in sites where the sealant was assessed as being completely lost. The final report of the trial, five years after placement of the sealant, showed that 56 per cent of treated sites retained sealant (Horowitz et al. 1977). This resulted in a 92 per cent prevention of dental caries in sites with retention of material.

Table 3. Nuva-Seal.

Time since application (years)	Complete retention (per cent)	Caries reduction (per cent)
1	88	81
2	73	67

Data from Horowitz et al. (1974).

NIDR Trial

In 1975 Stiles presented the results (some interim) of clinical trials with Nuva-Seal, supported by the National Caries Programme (NIDR). The studies, which investigated various aspects of sealant usage, included about 3,500 children. Most children were between six and 14 years of age. Application of the sealant was carried out by dentists, dental hygienists, dental assistants, dental corpsmen and public dental technicians or aides. The main findings of all six trials are summarized in Table 4. One must be cautious, however, in comparing these findings because each study was designed somewhat differently in an attempt to answer different aspects of the problem. It is obvious from the results that although the same material was used in each study, using the same application

Table 4. Nuva-Seal retention.

Study number	Fluorid-ated	Overall retention[1]					
		6 months (per cent)	12 months (per cent)	18 months (per cent)	24 months (per cent)	30 months (per cent)	48 months (per cent)
1	Yes	66	49				
2	Yes	39	16	8			
3	Yes		83		65		
4	No			51		39	
5	No		32		17	8 (36 m)	
6	No				84		66

[1] Data from Stiles (1975).

techniques, there is a great variation. The reasons for this may be twofold.

First, retention rates of sealant were based on the ability of the examiner to detect the material on the occlusal surface. The statement was made in the paper that the results 'would not reflect sealant limited to pit and fissure areas not accessible to examination with an explorer'. Thus, many regions containing sealant may not have been detected according to the examining criteria used and the ability of the examiner. Second, the wide range in the results could reflect differences in the application technique. Although the clinical technique is a quick and relatively simple one, there are critical stages. Moisture control after acid etching the occlusal surfaces, and their subsequent washing and drying, is critical before application of the resin and its polymerization. Several workers have shown the importance of the etching regimen in clinical bonding techniques. It is essential to prevent saliva from contaminating the etched surface before application of the resin. Thus, poor rates of retention in two of the studies shown in Table 4 are most likely caused by failure in the application technique, probably by salivary contamination of acid-etched surfaces before application of resin. Difficulty in detecting the resin on the occlusal surface during subsequent examination would further highlight the failure in retention of the material.

UK Trials

In the UK, several clinical trials using a number of fissure sealants have been carried out by Rock. In 1974 he reported the results of two years' work on four commercial sealants (Rock 1974). Each

Table 5. Nuva-Seal retention.

Time since application (months)	Full retention (per cent)	Partial retention (per cent)	Sealant lost (per cent)
6	91.1	7.2	1.7
12	86.2	10.3	3.5
24	80.0	15.3	4.7

Data from Rock (1974).

sealant was applied to two teeth in the mouths of 100 children between 11 and 13 years of age. The teeth sealed were in diagonally opposite quadrants, and teeth on the opposite side of each arch served as matched contralateral controls. The results after two years with Nuva-Seal are shown in Table 5. The material was fully intact on 80 per cent of teeth, and had produced an 89 per cent reduction in occlusal caries relative to controls. In addition, a further 15.3 per cent of teeth were classed as showing partial retention. Of the 170 teeth used in this aspect of the trial, only five teeth (2.9 per cent) in the test group showed evidence of occlusal caries two years after the initial application of the sealant. However, 49 of the control teeth (28.8 per cent) were carious (Table 6). One feature of relevance is that the numbers of teeth remaining fully sealed after two years were very similar to the numbers retaining sealant six months after application. This indicates that if the sealant is to be lost, it is lost early on, probably as a result of an incorrect application technique or polymerization failure, rather than failure of the sealant/enamel bond.

Table 6. Nuva-Seal: incidence of occlusal caries.

Time since application (years)	No. of teeth in study	Caries	
		Test teeth	Control teeth
2	170	5 (2.9%)	49 (28.8%)

Data from Rock (1974).

A previous trial with Nuva-Seal resin in combination with the Spectroline Lamp (Rock 1972) reported less satisfactory results (Table 7). However, when comparing the results of using the same material, applied by the same operator, but this time using the Nuva-Lite (Figure 54a and b) a significant difference in rates of retention between the two groups was seen (Table 7). This must be due to the more efficient polymerization of the sealant when using the intraoral Nuva-Lite, relative to the extraoral Spectroline lamp. It is interesting to note that in both groups there is little difference between the six-month and 12-month results. Once again, this

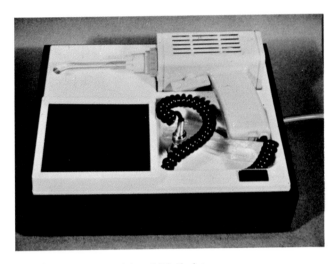

Figure 54a. *The Nuva-Lite UV light gun.*

infers that when the sealant is applied correctly and polymerized well in situ, it will remain in place. If it is to be lost this will occur early on in the trial.

In a Nuva-Seal study by Burt et al. (1975), 205 children between five and 17 years of age participated initially. Between them, 427 pairs of teeth were included in the study, one of each pair being sealed. At six months, 39 per cent of all teeth were graded as having the sealant completely intact, with a further 44.2 per cent classed as showing partial retention. However, the total retention figure of 83.2 per cent may be the significant one with regard to prevention of caries as a result of partial loss of sealant, which usually occurs on cuspal slopes. This may not reduce the efficacy of the seal.

Douglas and Tranter (1975) reported on a two-year study using Nuva-Seal in the Aberdare region of South Wales. The age range of the 106 patients was six to 13 years, presenting a complete spectrum of the mixed dentition. Of the 275 teeth sealed in the study, 86.2 per cent were found to be fully sealed after two years, with 6.2 per cent showing partial retention, while 7.6 per cent showed loss of sealant (Table 8). Regarding caries incidence, 9.1

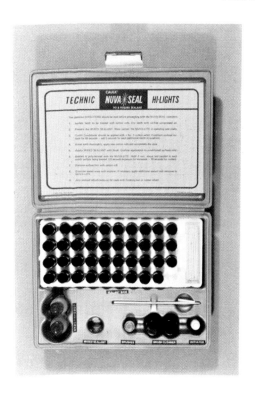

Figure 54b. *Nuva-Seal fissure sealant kit.*

Table 7. Nuva-Seal retention.

	Time since application (months)	Retention (per cent)		Total retention
		Complete	Partial	
Spectroline lamp plus Nuva-Seal	6	56	26	82
	12	54	24	78
Nuva-Lite	6	91	7	98
	12	86	10	96

Data from Rock (1972).

Table 8. Nuva-Seal retention.

No. of teeth	Time since application (months)	Full retention (per cent)	Partial retention (per cent)	Sealant lost (per cent)
275	24	86.2	6.2	7.6

Data from Douglas and Tranter (1975).

per cent of test teeth were classed as being carious, whereas 36 per cent of controls became carious over the two-year period (Table 9). Nuva-Seal has recently been modified to form a second generation occlusal sealant, renamed Nuva-Cote. Nuva-Cote sealant is pre-activated, meaning that it is supplied ready mixed and it has a one-year shelf life. The filler used in Nuva-Cote produces a material with increased abrasion resistance relative to unfilled sealants. In addition, a new bulb assembly for the Nuva-lite has a shorter warm-up period and burns cooler so that the apparatus does not cut out as readily as the previous generation of Nuva-lites.

Epoxylite 9075

When Epoxylite 9075 was used by Rock (1974), he showed that two years after application, 51.5 per cent of the fissures exhibited full retention of the sealant, with a further 15.0 per cent showing partial retention (Table 10). In this aspect of the trial 167 teeth were used. However, when the incidence of occlusal caries is examined (Table 11) only nine teeth (5.4 per cent) in the test group developed occlusal caries, despite the fact that only 51.5 per cent of the test teeth were classed as being fully sealed. In the controls, 58 teeth (34.7 per cent) showed occlusal caries. This finding suggests

Table 9. Nuva-Seal: incidence of occlusal caries.

No. of teeth	Carious test teeth	Carious control teeth
274	25 (9.1%)	99 (36.0%)

Data from Douglas and Tranter (1975).

Table 10. Epoxylite 9075 retention.

Time since application (months)	Full retention (per cent)	Partial retention (per cent)	Sealant lost (per cent)
6	58.6	18.8	22.6
12	52.6	18.7	28.7
24	51.5	15.0	33.5

Data from Rock (1974).

that more of the sealant remained on teeth in the test group than was clinically detectable. This resin has a very low viscosity before polymerization, which may allow it to penetrate more efficiently into narrow fissures than other resins as shown by in vitro studies (Silverstone 1974).

Table 11. Epoxylite 9075: incidence of occlusal caries.

Time since application (years)	No. of teeth in study	Caries	
		Test teeth	Control teeth
2	167	9 (5.4%)	58 (34.7%)

Data from Rock (1974).

Concise and Delton

Two chemically polymerized Bis-GMA sealants are currently available and have produced good results in vitro and in vivo. Concise Enamel Bond System (3M Dental Products, St Paul, Minn.) and Delton (Johnson and Johnson, New Jersey) are fairly similar resins, the former being supplied with 37 per cent phosphoric acid as the etching agent whilst the latter employs a 35 per cent solution of phosphoric acid. The clinical effectiveness of Delton fissure sealant after one year was reported by Houpt and Sheykholeslam (1978). Two hundred and five subjects, aged between six and ten years, that had a pair of caries-free contralateral first permanent molars were selected. After 11 months, 185 children were re-examined. Only five of the treated teeth showed

107

evidence of caries, whereas 53 of the control molars were carious. The sealant was assessed as being 90 per cent effective in preventing dental caries.

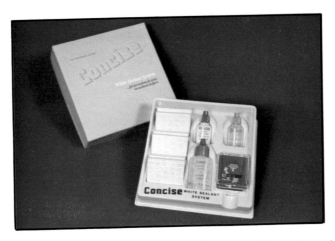

Figure 55. *Concise White Sealant System. This chemically polymerized resin has a brilliant white colour to aid in its clinical detection.*

Following application of Concise Enamel Bond sealant, 60 per cent of the sealants were present after two years (Thylstrup and Poulsen 1978). The effectivenes of the treatment was highly significant, the caries reduction being about 50 per cent overall, irrespective of sealant status. Where the material was fully retained, caries reduction was 98 per cent.

A new version of the 3M product has been introduced recently. Named 'Concise White Sealant System' (Figure 55) it is essentially the same as its forerunner with the addition of a titanium salt to give the resin a brilliant white colour. Simonsen (1978) has carried out studies on Concise White Sealant System and has published findings 12 months after application. A total of 583 permanent and 436 deciduous teeth were sealed initially. At 12 months, 96 per cent of the permanent teeth retained sealant whereas 98.9 per cent retention was found with deciduous teeth. Initial examination of the patients at two years indicates relatively little change compared

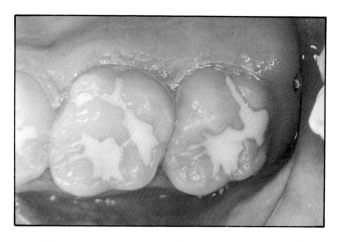

Figure 56a. *Teeth sealed with 3M Concise White Sealant seen six months after application. The brilliant white colour contrasts with tooth colour.*

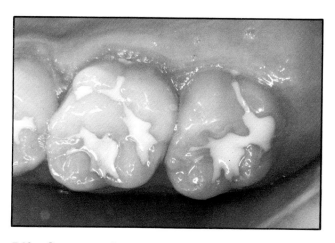

Figure 56b. *Same patient as in Figure 56a seen 18 months after placement of the sealant. There appears to be little difference between this and the six month result, demonstrating the efficacy of the seal and the ease of detection of the resin.*

with the one year result (Simonsen 1978, pers. comm.). Figure 56a is one of the cases in the trial by Simonsen showing the white sealant in places six months after application. The brilliant white colour contrasts with tooth colour and the resin is easily detectable. Figure 56b shows the same case 18 months after application, demonstrating the efficacy of the seal and the ease of detection of the resin.

Alpha-Seal

Alpha-Seal was also tested in the clinical trial by Rock (1974). The resin is polymerized by UV light using the Alpha-Lite (Amalgamated Dental Co., London), in which the UV beam is directed along a flexible quartz fibre-optic light guide (Figure 57, a and b). The sealant has a small quantity of Tinopal dye incorporated which fluoresces blue in UV light. The etching fluid supplied with the sealant is 30 per cent unbuffered phosphoric acid. This was selected in preference to 50 per cent buffered phosphoric acid after the work of Silverstone (1974) in which several etching agents were tested, together with phosphoric acid in the concentration range 20 to 70 per cent.

Rock (1977) has reported on his three year trial with Alpha-Seal. Three years after application of the resin on 180 permanent teeth, 70 per cent showed full retention of sealant with a further 22.3 per cent showing partial retention of the material (Table 12). Sealant loss was recorded in 7.7 per cent of the sample. The amount of new occlusal caries found on test and control teeth after three years is shown in Table 13. A highly significant caries reduction was demonstrated between test and contralateral control teeth. Clinically the new Alpha-Lite is easy and pleasant to use because only the nozzle of the fibre-optic is guided into the patient's mouth. The light guide is sheathed throughout its length so that the radiation is emitted only from the tip and, because no heat is involved or transmitted in this part of the apparatus, a cold beam is used. The material polymerizes in 20 seconds exposure to the UV beam, and the machine is ready for use within three minutes of switching on, irrespective of how long it has been used before switching off the apparatus.

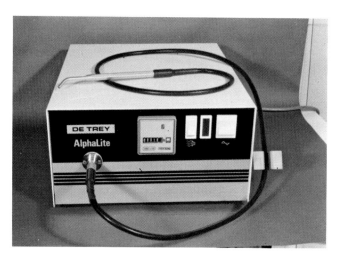

Figure 57a. *The Alpha-Lite UV light apparatus containing a quartz fibre-optic light guide.*

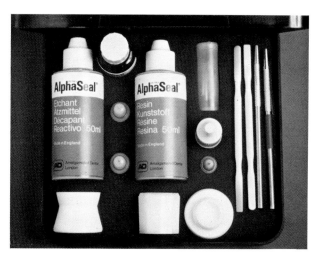

Figure 57b. *Alpha-Seal fissure sealant kit.*

New Ultraviolet Light Systems

Since 1977 two new UV light polymerizing systems have been

111

introduced. The Lee UV Curing Light System (Lee Pharmaceuticals, South El Monte, CA) employs a flexible lead to deliver UV light at wavelengths greater than 320 nm to the tooth surface. The sealant produced by this company is called Lee-Bond. A similar system has also been introduced by Kulzer, distributed by the Degussa Corporation (Placentia, CA). The UV light unit is known as Duralux UV-300, and has a similar flexible light conductor. The sealant is called Estilux glaze, and a UV-curing composite is also available. Both of these systems have only just been introduced and therefore there are no clinical trial figures available. The author has used both systems and is especially impressed by the UV delivery systems.

Table 12. Alpha-Seal retention.

Time since application (months)	Full retention (per cent)	Partial retention (per cent)	Sealant lost (per cent)
6	90.0	9.4	0.6
12	82.0	12.9	5.1
36	70.0	22.3	7.7

Data from Rock (1977).

Results of Trials

It has been stated that application of an occlusal sealant does not protect against approximal caries. However, to criticize fissure sealants on the basis that approximal caries reduces their value is to condemn a valuable caries preventive measure in isolation. In

Table 13. Alpha-Seal: incidence of occlusal caries.

Time since application (years)	No. of teeth in study	Caries	
		Test teeth	Control teeth
1	178	4	26
3	161	11	34

Data from Rock (1977).

areas with low fluoride levels in the public water supplies, the application of sealant should always be accompanied by a topical fluoride regimen, in one form or another.

Thus, the results of many trials in various parts of the world have shown that fissure sealants can have a highly significant effect in the prevention of occlusal caries. Most studies have shown that the UV-activated materials produce the most satisfactory, and reproducible, results. However, it is also evident that more attention must be paid to the application technique if the materials are to be highly effective in everyone's hands. Perhaps it is because the application technique is so simple and quick to carry out that not enough attention has been paid to detail. These materials have also been tested in a private practice environment. Doyle and Brose (1978) carried out a study using Nuva-Seal in their orthodontic practice for a five-year period. A total of 428 patients participated in the study, at the conclusion of which 92 per cent of permanent teeth retained sealant. This demonstrates the important part sealants can play in caries prevention in the dental office.

Technique of Fissure Sealing

The technique of fissure sealing is one in which the vulnerable biting surfaces of teeth are coated with a thin layer of a plastic-type material to prevent the initiation and progress of caries. The technique consists essentially of two stages: 'conditioning' of the tooth surface (using an acid solution), and application of the sealant.

The use of an acid solution to etch the enamel surface is an essential prerequisite for the successful bonding of resin to the hard tissue. The acid usually employed is phosphoric acid with an exposure time of 60 seconds. Buonocore (1955) used 85 per cent phosphoric acid solution to etch or 'condition' enamel prior to the use of acrylic restorative materials in order to improve the edge adaptation. Since then, many workers have used a solution of 50 per cent phosphoric acid, buffered with seven per cent zinc oxide by weight, as an etching agent prior to bonding of sealants or composite resins to enamel.

It has been shown that the acid solution produces changes to the enamel surface in two distinct ways (Silverstone 1974). In the first, a shallow layer of enamel, approximately $10\,\mu m$ in depth, is removed by etching (Figure 58). In this manner plaque, surface and subsurface pellicles are effectively removed from the site to be bonded. In addition, chemically inert crystals in surface enamel are also removed, so favouring attempts at chemical union between hard tissue and resin. In the second, after removal of the surface layer by etching, the remaining enamel surface is rendered porous by the acid solution (Figure 59). It is into this porous region that the resin is able to penetrate and so bond with the enamel. The depth of enamel rendered porous can be measured accurately in polarized light (Silverstone 1974). Electron-microscopic examination of the enamel/resin junction shows that an excellent bond occurs between enamel and resin, irrespective of the material used (Figure 60). The most important parameter is to obtain a satisfactory initial etch. Demineralization of enamel to reveal the fitting resin surface demonstrates the extent of penetration of the resin into etched enamel. Tags of up to $50\,\mu m$ in length are identified routinely (Figures 61 and 62) and present a formidable area for retention.

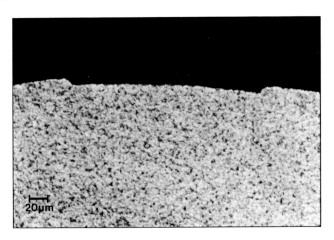

Figure 58. *Longitudinal ground section showing a region of enamel exposed to 30 per cent phosphoric acid for 60 seconds examined in water between crossed polars. A layer of enamel measuring 10 μm has been removed from the window region by etching.*

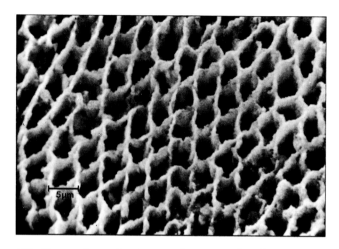

Figure 59. *Scanning electron micrograph of an enamel surface which has been etched with phosphoric acid for 60 seconds. The etch pattern is one in which prism centres have been removed preferentially, termed a Type 1 etching pattern.*

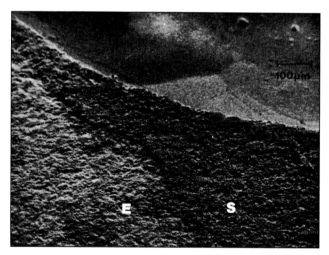

Figure 60. *Examination of the enamel—sealant junction with the scanning electron microscope shows no evidence of separation of the sealant (S) from the enamel (E), in spite of section preparation and examination procedures.*

115

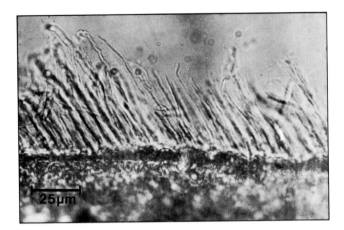

Figure 61. *The enamel—sealant junction can be exposed by complete demineralization of enamel. The fitting surface of the sealant shows a row of tags which had previously penetrated the etched enamel surface. Tag lengths vary from 25 to 50 μm.*

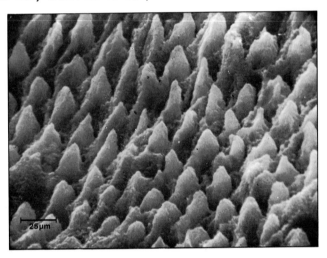

Figure 62. *Scanning electron micrograph of another sample of fissure sealant (3M Enamel Bond) after demineralization of the adjacent enamel. The inner fitting surface of the resin shows tags which are approximately 30 μm in length.*

116

Range of Etchants and Solutions

Many studies have been carried out with a 50 per cent solution of phosphoric acid buffered with seven per cent zinc oxide by weight (Buonocore et al. 1968; Gwinnett 1967). However, in a recent study (Silverstone 1974) a number of different acid solutions, as well as phosphoric acid in the concentration range 20 to 70 per cent, were investigated for their effects on enamel surfaces in vitro. Phosphoric acid was found to be the most successful agent for etching enamel surfaces prior to application of a resin. The degree of etching increased with decreasing acid concentration (Figure 63).

The most retentive conditions for a sealant were found to be in the range 20 to 50 per cent, with a 30 per cent (w/w) unbuffered solution of phosphoric acid being the most effective single agent.

In a further study (Silverstone 1975) phosphoric acid solutions in the concentration range 5 to 80 per cent (w/w) were investigated for their effects on human enamel surfaces, with special reference to the variation in degree of etching over single tooth surfaces. When using acid concentrations of 5 to 15 per cent and 70 to 80 per cent, only minimal surface changes were found (Figures 64 and 65). The most evenly distributed etching patterns were found with solutions of 30 to 40 per cent phosphoric acid used with 60 second exposure periods. A 30 per cent unbuffered solution of phosphoric acid produced the most consistent and evenly distributed etch over a single enamel surface.

Types of Etching Patterns

Silverstone et al, (1975) found three basic etching patterns when human dental enamel was exposed to phosphoric acid.

Type 1

In Type 1 etching pattern there was a generalized roughening of the enamel surface, but with a distinct pattern showing hollowing of prism centres with relatively intact peripheral regions (Figure 59). The average diameter of the hollowed regions was 3 μm. This was found to be the most common of the three patterns observed.

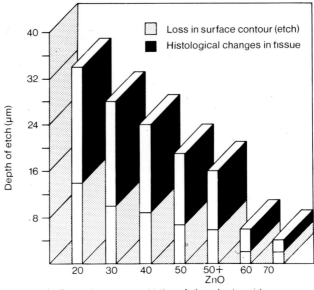

Figure 63. *Histogram showing the depth of enamel affected by 60-second exposure to various concentrations of phosphoric acid. This consists of both loss in depth due to etching and the region showing histological change due to the creation of porous regions.*

Type 2

In Type 2 etching pattern, prism peripheries appeared to be removed, or heavily damaged (Figure 66). Therefore, the prism cores were left projecting towards the original enamel surface. This damage of the peripheral regions of the prisms was seen to extend along the length of the prism, thus aiding in delineating individual prisms. When viewed from the original surface, separate bundles or columns of material were seen, the gaps separating them corresponding to the peripheral regions of the prisms. Thus, this Type 2 etching pattern is the reverse of the honeycomb pattern of Type 1

118

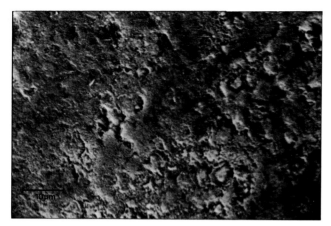

Figure 64. *Scanning electron micrograph of an enamel surface which has been etched for 60 seconds with 10 per cent phosphoric acid. While many regions of the surface appear uneven, with evidence of pitting, large areas are indistinguishable from sound enamel.*

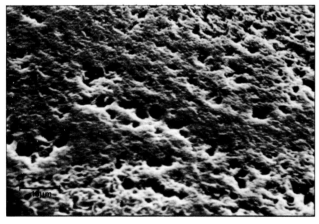

Figure 65. *Scanning electron micrograph of an enamel surface which was etched for 60 seconds with 70 per cent phosphoric acid. Although there is some pitting, the surface shows relatively little evidence of acid attack, appearing similar to specimens which were exposed to 10 per cent phosphoric acid.*

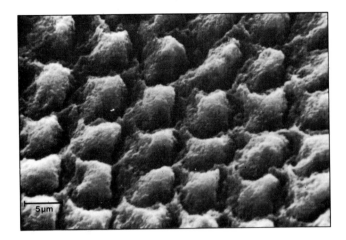

Figure 66. *Scanning electron micrograph of an enamel surface which has been exposed to 40 per cent phosphoric acid for 60 seconds. In this case the etching pattern is one in which there has been a preferential removal of prism peripheries, termed a Type 2 etching pattern.*

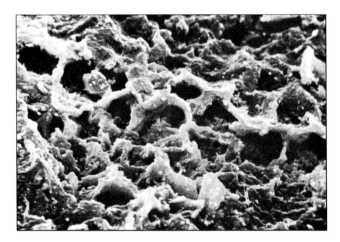

Figure 67. *Scanning electron micrograph of an enamel surface treated with 30 per cent phosphoric acid for 60 seconds. The etching pattern shows a generalized surface roughening with no apparent evidence of a prism pattern. Such surfaces are referred to as a Type 3 etching pattern.*

120

damage, and both patterns are produced by exposure to a similar solution of phosphoric acid for an identical exposure time.

Type 3

Some etched regions showed neither Type 1 nor Type 2 etching patterns exclusively. These areas appeared as a generalized surface roughening, referred to as a Type 3 etching pattern (Figure 67). The whole region in the Type 3 etching pattern was one in which the surface topography could not be related to a prism pattern. All three patterns of etching were found to occur on the one enamel surface, produced by identical conditions of acid attack. This highlights the variation in structure that can occur in enamel, not only from tooth to tooth or surface to surface, but also from site to site on a single tooth surface.

Etching Patterns in Deciduous Teeth

When employing deciduous enamel it was necessary to etch the surface for 120 seconds in order to produce etching patterns comparable to those found in permanent enamel. Several workers have recorded the presence of areas of prismless enamel on the surface of deciduous teeth. However, not all studies are in agreement with respect to its prevalence. In the studies by Ripa (1966) and Ripa et al. (1966), prismless enamel was found to occur in 100 per cent of their samples of deciduous enamel. Studies by Buonocore (1971) and Ripa and Cole (1970) have shown better retention rates of fissure sealants in permanent than in deciduous teeth. The existence of the prismless layer on deciduous enamel is thus thought to prevent the penetration of resins into the enamel surface even after etching with phosphoric acid (Sheykholeslam and Buonocore 1972). In a more recent study (Hinding and Sveen 1974) a lesser degree of dissolution of occlusal surfaces was found with deciduous enamel than with permanent enamel after etching with phosphoric acid. These workers too concluded that this might be related to the presence of prismless enamel in the surface of deciduous teeth.

Horsted et al. (1976) compared enamel structure and crystal orientation on occlusal surfaces in deciduous and permanent teeth. In contrast to the studies just quoted, however, these workers concluded that only on rare occasions was prismless surface enamel observed. The main crystal orientation and prism arrangement was found to be identical in deciduous and permanent enamel. Similarly, in a previous study in which 100 carious lesions in deciduous enamel were examined histologically (Silverstone 1970), only 17 per cent of the material showed evidence of areas of prismless enamel. Such regions of prismless enamel were found to occur most commonly in the cervical region of the tooth, and not on the occlusal surface. Thus, poor retention of fissure sealants on deciduous enamel cannot be attributed wholly to the presence of areas of prismless enamel, in view of the differences in findings with respect to its prevalence and significance.

In the studies by Silverstone (1975) and Silverstone and Dogon (1976), a 60 second etch with phosphoric acid in the concentration range 20 to 50 per cent did not produce etching patterns or degrees of porosity comparable to those seen in permanent enamel. Under these conditions deciduous enamel surfaces were etched poorly, with many regions showing little evidence of surface porosity. However, when the etching time was increased, more convincing etching patterns were produced (Figure 68). With 30 per cent phosphoric acid, an exposure period of 120 seconds produced etching patterns which were more or less comparable to those seen in permanent enamel. Whilst there is little doubt now that a well marked prism pattern can be produced on occlusal surfaces of deciduous teeth, there still remains the question as to why a prolonged etching time is necessary. As a result of its lower mineral content and higher internal pore volume, erupted deciduous surface enamel is likely to contain larger amounts of exogenous organic material than permanent surface enamel. This factor may be an extremely important one in deciding the etching characteristics of deciduous surface enamel and may be the explanation, in part at least, for the necessity for a longer etching time to produce surface damage comparable to that found in permanent enamel.

Has There Been Etching-Related Caries?

No evidence of caries or demineralization of test teeth has been reported which could be related to the original etching of the

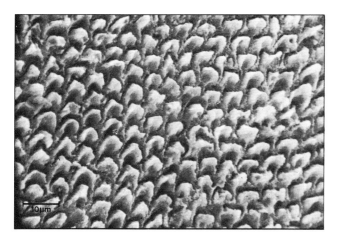

Figure 68. *Scanning electron micrograph of part of the occlusal enamel from a deciduous molar tooth which had been etched for 120 seconds with 30 per cent phosphoric acid. The surface shows a convincing pattern of etched prism exhibiting a Type 2 etching pattern. There is no evidence of prismless enamel.*

enamel. Acid etching is an essential stage in the bonding mechanism and it appears to be confined to the cuspal slopes, rather than to the base of the fissure, and this is the region where the bond occurs (Gwinnett and Buonocore 1972; Silverstone 1974). In addition, a number of studies have shown that etched enamel, not covered by resin, will be remineralized on contact with the oral fluid (Albert and Grenoble 1971; Silverstone 1973). Quantitative studies on enamel solubility rates have shown recently that the solubility rate of acid etched enamel returns to that of adjacent sound enamel after 24 hours of exposure to oral fluid (Silverstone 1977). In addition, fissure sealed enamel surfaces artificially abraded in vitro show a lower solubility rate than adjacent sound enamel (Silverstone 1977). These results were interpreted as being due to the retention of tags of sealant, which penetrated up to 50 μm into the enamel surface. Thus, fissure sealed enamel surfaces which have been worn down might well be less susceptible to caries than adjacent sound enamel.

Preventive Dentistry

Acid Etching: Clinical Technique

Since the acid etching regimen is so important in the clinical application of fissure sealants, it is relevant to describe the clinical technique in some detail. Identical principles should be adopted for any acid etch procedure, especially since the acid etch technique is used extensively in restorative and other branches of dentistry.

Step 1

Carry out a routine dental prophylaxis so that enamel surfaces to be fissure sealed are cleaned thoroughly. It is important to use a prophylaxis paste that is free from glycerine and fluoride ions. With the former, an impervious coating can be laid down on the enamel surface, whereas with the latter the enamel will be more difficult to etch. After prophylaxis, wash away remains of paste and oral debris.

Step 2

Sealant should be applied to teeth in one quadrant of the mouth at a time. Isolate the quadrant using cotton wool rolls and a saliva ejector in conjunction with an efficient high speed aspirator. For sealing mandibular teeth a flanged saliva ejector is desirable to prevent interference from the tongue. The use of a rubber dam is highly desirable but not absolutely essential.

Step 3

Dry the teeth to be sealed. Apply acid etching fluid to occlusal surfaces of the relevant teeth using a small brush. A sable-hair brush, gauge 00, is ideal (Figure 69). Leave the acid solution on the occlusal surfaces for 60 seconds. The occlusal surface and approximately halfway up the cuspal slopes should be etched. Gently rub the brush over the occlusal surface from time to time. Gentle agitation of the acid solution in this manner will increase dissolution phenomena, resulting in an even etch over the entire surface covered by the acid. The use of acid-soaked cotton pledgets

124

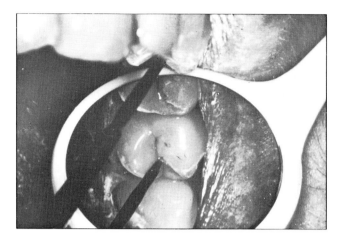

Figure 69. *The use of a sable-hair brush to carry the etchant to the occlusal surfaces. In this manner the acid can be placed accurately on to relevant tooth surfaces without the danger of spilling on to the soft tissues. Gentle agitation of the acid with the brush will result in an even etch of the surfaces treated.*

for etching is disliked by the author for several reasons. A pledget will absorb a large volume of acid solution so that, on rubbing over an occlusal surface, acid may run down buccal and lingual surfaces to contact the gingival margin. The use of a fine brush is more accurate in location of acid on the tooth surface. In addition, the fine tip of the brush will place acid into the fissure orifice. With a cotton pledget, air bubbles can be trapped in the fissure on application of the pledget.

Step 4

After 60 seconds, wash off the acid solution with water from an air/water triple spray syringe. It is not necessary to flood the patient's mouth. A steady stream of water/compressed air for approximately 5 seconds is adequate. Immediately dry the teeth in the relevant quadrant with compressed air from the triple spray.

125

Replace the cotton wool rolls at this stage. Continue with compressed air until all moisture has been removed from the occlusal surfaces. If the acid etching regimen is successful, the surface will appear 'frosted white'. If not, repeat the etching stage again.

Step 5

At this stage it is essential that no saliva be allowed to contaminate the etched enamel surface. This is probably the most important phase in the technique. If saliva is allowed to come into contact with the etched enamel surface, a very poor bond, or no bond at all, will result. If contamination occurs, repeat the 60 second etching cycle.

Step 6

Apply the mixed fissure sealant to all etched surfaces in the quadrant using a sable-hair brush. A brush similar to that used for acid etching is ideal. However, employ a colour-coded system to distinguish between brushes. If UV light is used, polymerize each occlusal surface for the required time. Rather than use the manufacturer's recommended exposure time, experiment with a small drop of sealant before use so that the operator will have confidence in the exposure times employed. Not only do current UV machines vary in their output, they also become less effective in time due to deposits occurring on the UV lamp. If the sealant is an auto-polymerized one, use the manufacturer's recommended exposure time, since this is more likely to be controlled. However, it is a sound policy to test the setting time in vitro before using it in vivo. Most chemically cured sealants require approximately 60 seconds.

Step 7

After polymerization, a blunt explorer should be used to feel gently over the entire sealant layer. Do not press hard on the explorer as if attempting to diagnose caries. Ideally, an instrument such as a 'Thymozin' (Figure 70) should be employed. This is identical to an explorer with the exception that the end finishes as a small ball-ended burnisher instead of a point. The sealed surface should feel completely smooth. If a deficiency is found, more sealant should be applied. There is likely to be an 'air inhibited' sticky layer on the surface of the polymerized sealant. This is sometimes diagnosed incorrectly as incomplete polymerization of the sealant. This layer should be wiped off the sealant using pledgets of cotton wool.

Step 8

It is very important to check that the air line to the air/water triple spray is not contaminated with water or oil vapour. If this occurs, a fine layer of moisture and/or oil will be deposited on to the etched surface and will certainly prevent the sealant bonding to the hard tissue. The air line should be checked by blowing compressed air from the air/water triple spray on to a plane mirror. If the air line is contaminated, this will show as droplets of water and/or oil forming on the surface of the mirror after 30 to 60 seconds.

Other Uses of Acid Etching

In addition to its use in the primary prevention of occlusal caries, the acid etch technique is now used extensively in other branches of dentistry. The composite restorative materials are, in essence, filled sealants. Thus, a composite material can be bonded directly on to acid etched enamel. In this manner, unfilled resin will penetrate etched enamel while the filled resin will be maintained in place by the large number of tags formed. Some manufacturers advise coating the etched enamel surface with a layer of unfilled resin (sealant) first, followed by application of the filled resin. Most evidence suggests that this results in a better bond with the etched enamel surface, so reducing the possibility of microleakage and loss of the restoration (Dogon 1975).

Perhaps the greatest impact in restorative dentistry has been the restoration of fractured incisor teeth in young children. This has always presented a problem for the paedodontist, who has had to use techniques such as basket crowns and, in more recent years, open-faced stainless steel crowns. Using the acid etch technique, fractured incisors can now be restored with composite materials,

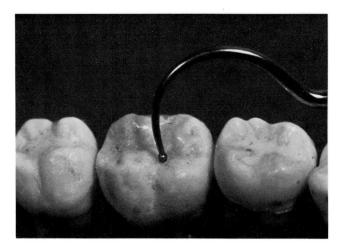

Figure 70. *The use of a Thymozin instrument will detect any sealant deficiencies, if they exist, without damaging the newly polymerized resin.*

producing excellent results. Such restorations last many years and are aesthetically good (Figure 71). A number of reports have been published in many parts of the world demonstrating the significance and stability of such restorations. The technique can also be used to mask hypoplastic and stained teeth. Since the main mechanism of attachment of the restorative material is due to mechanical bonding, only minimal preparation of a tooth surface need be carried out. If the tooth, or teeth, to be restored are grossly discoloured, then it will be necessary to add a masking agent to the composite material (Figure 72).

The direct bonding technique has also made a significant contribution in orthodontics, where plastic or metal brackets can be bonded directly on to buccal enamel surfaces. Eliminating the necessity for bands not only results in a marked improvement in aesthetics, but also reduces the risk of demineralization of enamel under bands.

Conclusion

The overall contribution of the acid etch technique to dentistry has

128

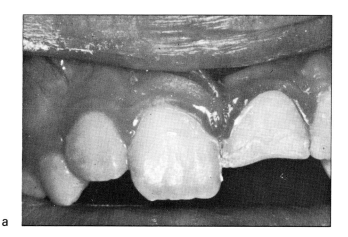

a

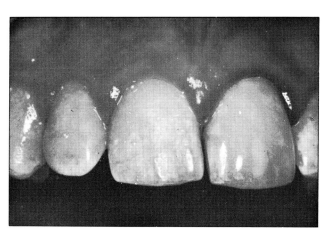

b

Figure 71. *(a) After trauma an eight-year-old girl had damaged her left maxillary central incisor, resulting in a horizontal fracture. (b) Same patient after restoration of the fractured incisor tooth with a composite material using the acid etch technique. This clinical photograph was taken three years after restoration. Opaque markings had been placed into the composite for aesthetic reasons. The gingival margin in relation to the restoration appears slightly swollen. This was due to prophylaxis carried out prior to photography so that the composite restoration could be reglazed.*

129

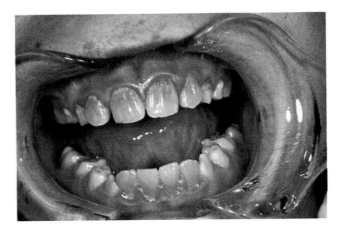

a

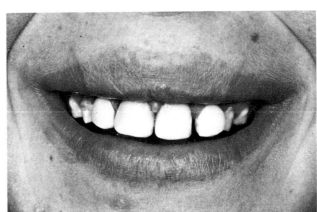

b

Figure 72. *(a) Clinical appearance of a young male with severe tetracycline-stained teeth. The patient was extremely self-conscious of his appearance. (b) Same patient after restoration of the anterior teeth with a composite material using the acid etch technique. Since the tetracycline discoloration is related to the dentine, it is necessary to add a white opaquer to the composite material to disguise the dark colour. Restoration such as these serve as an excellent temporary measure. If the patient is to have porcelain jacket crowns (or similar restorations) at a later date, the acid etch restoration in no way prejudices further treatment.*

been highly significant. The use of fissure sealants can reduce the incidence of occlusal caries drastically. Since occlusal caries accounts for approximately 50 per cent of the total caries experience, and since the occlusal site is least benefited by fluoride, fissure sealants play an important part in an overall caries preventive regimen.

References

Albert, M. and Grenoble, O. E., *J. S. Calif. Dent. Assoc.*, 1971, **39**, 747.

Ast, D. B., Bushel, A. and Chase, H. C., *J. Am. Dent. Assoc.*, 1950, **41**, 437.

Backer Dirks, O., Houwink, B. and Kwant, G. W., *Arch. Oral Biol.*, 1961, **5**, 284.

Bowen, R. L., U.S. Patent No. 3,066,122 (Nov. 1962).

Buonocore, M. G., *J. Dent. Res.*, 1955, **34**, 849.

Buonocore, M. G., *J. Am. Dent. Assoc.*, 1971, **82**, 1090.

Buonocore, M. G., Matsui, A. and Gwinnett, A. J., *Arch. Oral Biol.*, 1968, **13**, 61.

Burt, B., Berman, D. S., Gelbier, S. and Silverstone, L. M., *Br. Dent. J.*, 1975, **138**, 98.

Cameron, J. L., Woodward, S. C., Pulaski, E. J., Sleeman, K. H., Brandes, G., Kulkarni, R. K. and Leonard, F., *Surgery*, 1965, **58**, 424.

Crabb, J. J. and Wilson, H. J., *Dent. Practit.*, 1971, **22**, 111.

Cueto, A. and Buonocore, M. G., *J. Am. Dent. Assoc.*, 1967, **73**, 121.

Dogon, I. L., in *Proc. Int. Symp. Acid Etch Technique*, L. M. Silverstone and I. L. Dogon (Eds), pp. 100–118, North Central, Minnesota, 1975.

Douglas, W. H. and Tranter, T. C., *Proc. Br. Paediatr. Soc.*, 1975, **5**, 17.

Doyle, W. A. and Brose, J. A., *J. Dent. Child.*, 1978, **45**, 23.

Gwinnett, A. J., *Arch. Oral Biol.*, 1967, **12**, 1615.

Gwinnett, A. J. and Buonocore, M. G., *Arch. Oral Biol.*, 1972, **17**, 415.

Hinding, J. H. and Sveen, O. B., *Arch. Oral Biol.*, 1974, **19**, 573.

Horowitz, H. S., Heifetz, S. B. and McCune, R. J., *J. Am. Dent. Assoc.*, 1974, **89**, 885.

Horowitz, H. S., Heifetz, S. B. and Poulsen, S., *J. Am. Dent. Assoc.*, 1977, **95**, 1133.

Horsted, M., Fejerskov, O., Larsen, M. J. and Thylstrup, A., *Caries Res.*, 1976, **10**, 287.

Houpt, M. and Sheykholeslam, Z., *J. Dent. Child.*, 1978, **45**, 26.

Hyatt, T. P., *Dent. Cosmos*, 1923, **65**, 234.

Klein, H. and Knutson, J. W., *J. Am. Dent. Assoc.*, 1942, **29**, 1420.

McCune, R. J., Horowitz, H. S. and Heifetz, S. B., *J. Am. Dent Assoc.*, 1973, **87**, 1177.

Preventive Dentistry

Miller, J., *Br. Dent. J.*, 1950, **91**, 92.

Nathan, H. S., Nachlas, M. M., Solomon, R. D., Hapern, B. D. and Seligman, A. M., *Ann. Surg.*, 1960, **152**, 648.

Oswald, J., *J. Proc. 80th Health Congr. R. Soc. Health*, 1973, 71.

Parkhouse, R. C. and Winter, G. B., *Br. Dent. J.*, 1971, **130**, 16.

Ripa, L. W., *J. Dent. Res.*, 1966, **45**, 5.

Ripa, L. W. and Cole, W. W., *J. Dent. Res.*, 1970, **49**, 171.

Ripa, L. W., Gwinnett, A. J. and Buonocore, M. G., *Arch. Oral Biol.,* 1966, **11**, 41.

Rock, W. P., *Br. Dent. J.*, 1972, **133**, 146.

Rock, W. P., *Br. Dent. J.*, 1974, **136**, 317.

Rock, W. P., *Br. Dent. J.*, 1977, **142**, 16.

Roydhouse, R., *J. Dent. Child*, 1968, **35**, 253.

Sheykholeslam, Z. and Buonocore, M. G., *J. Dent. Res.*, 1972, **51**, 1572.

Silverstone, L. M., *J. Dent. Child.*, 1970, **37**, 17.

Silverstone, L. M., *Helv. Odont. Acta*, 1973, **17**, 64.

Silverstone, L. M., *Caries Res.*, 1974, **8**, 2.

Silverstone, L. M., in *Proc. Int. Symp. Acid Etch Technique*, L. M. Silverstone and I. L. Dogon (Eds), pp. 13–39, North Central, Minnesota, 1975.

Silverstone, L. M., *Caries Res.*, 1977, **11**, 46.

Silverstone, L. M. and Dogon, I. L., *J. Int. Assoc. Dent. Child.*, 1976, **7**, 11.

Silverstone, L. M., Saxton, C. A., Dogon, I. L. and Fejerskov, O., *Caries Res.*, 1975, **9**, 373.

Simonsen, R. J., *Clinical Applications of the Acid Etch Technique*, Quintessence, Chicago, 1978.

Stiles, H. M., in *Proc. Int. Symp. Acid Etch Technique*, L. M. Silverstone and I. L. Dogon (Eds), pp. 181–183, North Central, Minnesota, 1975.

Thylstrup, A. and Poulsen, S., *Scand. J. Dent. Res.*, 1978, **86**, 21.

8. Diet and Dental Caries

Dental caries is widespread amongst populations in technically developing nations and is rapidly approaching the severity levels found in affluent societies. The change in dietary habits associated with technical and economic development is most probably responsible for such a deterioration in dental health. The total food and drink intake, including non-nutrient components, is termed the diet. Dietary constituents come into contact with the teeth, their supporting tissues and with dental plaque. Thus the diet may exert a local effect on caries in the mouth by reacting with the enamel surface and by serving as a substrate for cariogenic micro-organisms. This chapter examines some of the evidence available on the relationship between diet and dental caries. In addition, the effects of the diet on dental plaque will be discussed as well as possible protective factors available in foodstuffs, and the replacement of sucrose by other sweeteners.

Epidemiological Evidence

A people whose natural diet is virtually free from fermentable carbohydrate are the Eskimos. The diet consists almost entirely of animal and fish protein and fat. Surveys have shown that Eskimo populations living in their natural habitat are virtually free from dental caries. However, when the Eskimos came into contact with trading stations and had access to a modern 'Western' diet, their dental caries experience rose drastically to be comparable with that of Western man. Thus, a marked increase in caries seems the inescapable result of the adoption of a modern 'civilized' diet. A well-defined case is that of the inhabitants of the island of Tristan da Cunha, an isolated group of people who lived for many years as subsistence farmers and fishermen. Their dental health was excellent when their diet comprised potatoes and other vegetables, meat and fish. The evacuation of the population to Britain in time of crisis was associated with an increase in dental caries experience which has continued since their return to the island. Tristan is probably the best example of dental deterioration associated with the consumption of sophisticated foods enjoyed by populations with an improved standard of living (Fisher 1972).

The dietary pattern in many countries was modified during World War II. The total consumption of carbohydrates was unchanged in the UK but there was a marked increase in the consumption of high extraction flours and a reduction in the consumption of sucrose. The most significant change was in the availability of sucrose for the manufacture of confectionery. These changes were accompanied by a decrease in dental caries experience in young children. This continued until sugar became readily available and rationing was finally abolished. Mellanby and Mellanby (1950) showed that the increased ease of obtaining sugar was associated with a rise in caries experience in children of comparable age groups. Similar findings were reported from Scandinavia (Toverud 1950) and Japan (Takeuchi 1961). The common factor in all these studies was the reduction in the consumption of easily fermentable carbohydrate, especially in the amount available for consumption between meals.

Mansbridge (1960), in a survey of over 400 Edinburgh schoolchildren aged 12 to 14 years, reported that those who consumed 8 oz of sweets and chocolate per week had a greater dental caries experience than those who consumed less than this amount.

In England, records of the past 100 years show a steady increase in the sucrose consumption from 20 lb per capita per annum in 1835 to 122 lb in 1961.

Dentists' Children

Ludwig and co-workers (1960) carried out a survey of the teeth of children of dental practitioners in New Zealand. It was found that children in the age group three to five years had an average of 0.9 decayed, extracted and filled (def) teeth. This compared with an average def of 6.3 in a control group of the same age range.

A study by Bradford and Crabb (1961) showed that a significant number of children of members of the dental profession had a controlled intake of refined carbohydrate. Two significant conclusions were drawn from the study. First, at any age from 5 to 11 years, the proportion of dentists' children who required no dental treatment of the deciduous dentition was twice that of the five-year-olds of the nation as a whole. Second, children of dentists who had decayed, extracted or filled deciduous teeth at ages from 5 to 11 years all required, or had received, less treatment than the nation's average five-year-olds.

Hereditary Fructose Intolerance

Hereditary fructose intolerance (HFI) is an uncommon metabolic disorder caused by an absence of hepatic fructose-1-phosphate aldolase, the enzyme which splits fructose-1-phosphate into two three-carbon fragments which are subsequently metabolized. HFI is characterized by nausea, vomiting, malaise, excessive sweating, tremor, coma and convulsions following the ingestion of foods containing fructose. Most of these symptoms can be attributed to a secondary hypoglycaemia which occurs after fructose ingestion.

Fructose occurs in the human diet in certain fruits (e.g. grapes) and vegetables, but by far the commonest source of fructose is sucrose. Patients suffering from this autosomal recessive genetic defect, if they survive early childhood, learn to avoid all forms of sweets, chocolates, candies, cakes, cookies and other sucrose-containing foods. One dental survey of HFI patients (Marthaler and Froesch 1967) involving patients of both sexes from 6 to 41 years of age, revealed 8 out of 19 individuals to be caries-free. This is in marked contrast to a random group where only one caries-free individual is generally found out of about 4,000 persons. In addition, the DMFT score of HFI patients who have decayed, missing or restored teeth is extremely low compared to the general population in an equivalent age group. Caries, if present at all, is restricted to occlusal fissures and is not found on smooth surfaces. Other members of the same families, who are not afflicted by HFI, show a caries experience comparable to that of the general population as a whole.

Evidence from the Regulation of Diet in Humans

The Vipeholm Study

In 1939, the Swedish Government requested the Royal Medical Board to investigate measures to reduce the frequency of the most common dental disease in Sweden, namely dental caries. This request led to a study of the relationship between diet and dental caries on 436 patients at the Vipeholm Mental Hospital in Lund (Gustafsson et al. 1959). The purpose of the study was to answer the following questions:

1. Does an increase in carbohydrate (mostly sugar) intake cause an increase in dental caries? If so, is caries actively influenced by: (a) the ingestion at meals of refined sugar in a non-sticky form; (b) the ingestion at meals of sugar in a sticky form; (c) the ingestion between meals of sugar in a sticky form?

2. Does a decrease in carbohydrate (sugar) intake produce a decrease in dental caries?

The main conclusions of the Vipeholm investigation were:

1. The risk of sugar increasing caries activity is great if the sugar is consumed in a form with a strong tendency to be retained on the surfaces of the teeth.

2. The risk of sugar increasing caries activity is greatest if the sugar is consumed between meals in a form which tends to be retained on the surfaces of the teeth with a transiently high concentration of sugar on these surfaces.

3. Increase in caries activity due to the intake of sugar-rich foodstuffs consumed in a manner favouring caries disappears on withdrawal of such foodstuffs from the diet.

4. Carious lesions may continue to appear despite the avoidance of refined sugar, maximum restriction of natural sugars and total

dietary carbohydrates.

5. The risk of an increase in caries activity is intensified with an increase in the duration of sugar clearance from the saliva.

6. A high sugar concentration in the saliva, in conjunction with a prolonged clearance time, increases caries activity.

Thus, the important fact emerged that the manner of administration and frequency of consumption were more closely related to subsequent development of dental caries than was the absolute amount of sugar consumed.

Other Studies

A thorough diet and dental caries study was carried out in Hopewood House, New South Wales, Australia. In this institutional study, sugar and white bread were virtually excluded from the diet. Carbohydrates were given in the form of wholemeal bread, soya beans, wheat germ, oats, rice, potatoes and some treacle and molasses. Dairy products, fruit, raw vegetables and nuts were eaten frequently. Although this was a vegetarian diet, it nevertheless provided an adequate amount of protein, fats, minerals and vitamins. In an early survey of Hopewood House children (Sullivan and Harris 1958) an extremely low caries prevalence was found. The water supply contained insignificant fluoride and the oral health of the children was poor. Thus, caries was reduced to a minimal level by dietary means alone. As the children grew older, they were relocated and therefore deviated from their original diet. In the period 1957 to 1961 a steep increase in DMFT experience occurred in the children above 13 years of age (Harris 1963). This indicated that the teeth had not acquired any permanent resistance to caries.

The Relative Cariogenicity of Carbohydrates

Many studies on the effect of diet on caries have been carried out in rats and other rodents. The basal diet of skimmed milk powder and dried liver was non-cariogenic in the experiments reported by Stephan (1966). Fruits, such as apples, which contain over 10 per cent of fermentable carbohydrates, cause caries and do not remove plaque or clean the teeth. Thus, finishing a meal with an apple is not a caries-preventive regimen as has been thought for many years. Grenby (1963) showed that when 66 per cent carbohydrate was incorporated into a skimmed milk–liver powder diet, sucrose was much more cariogenic than either glucose or raw wheat starch. Fructose has a cariogenicity score similar to glucose, and since these two sugars are the components of the sucrose molecule, it is evident that sucrose is much more cariogenic than its constituents. In many studies of relative cariogenicity sucrose has been found to be the most cariogenic. Presumably part of the special effect of sucrose is due to its ability to be converted into bacterial extracellular polysaccharides (e.g. dextran) which form part of the matrix of dental plaque. When starch solutions are applied to dental plaque no Stephan curve is seen. This may be because starch, being a polysaccharide, diffuses more slowly into plaque than mono- or disaccharides. Also, it is a polymer that must be hydrolyzed by extracellular amylase before it can be assimilated and metabolized by plaque bacteria.

Caries in Experimental Animals

Certain strains of rats and hamsters are susceptible to dental caries. In such animals diets containing 70 per cent of uncooked starches derived from wheat and maize are virtually non-cariogenic (Green and Hartles 1967). Diets containing 70 per cent sucrose instead of starch are highly cariogenic; a significant reduction in cariogenicity is only accomplished when the proportion of sucrose falls below 25 per cent (Green and Hartles 1969). Other sugars such as glucose, fructose, maltose, galactose and lactose are all highly cariogenic in the rat (Green and Hartles 1969). Research has indicated that sucrose is significantly more cariogenic than other simple sugars (Frostell et al. 1967; Grenby 1963; Guggenheim et al. 1966). Therefore, studies on the rat demonstrate that diets containing 70 per cent of one of the simple sugars are highly cariogenic but in some circumstances sucrose is the most cariogenic.

Animal studies therefore support the view that sucrose is the dietary component most likely to contribute to dental caries and more liable to promote caries than other sugars. Thus, the metabolism of sucrose by the microflora of the dental plaque differs from that of other sugars. If this is so, an understanding of these processes may be of importance in the dietary control of dental caries.

Diet and Dental Plaque

Seventy per cent of the plaque microflora are streptococci and they can all convert sugars into acids. With the introduction of gnotobiotic (germ-free) techniques to the study of dental caries, it soon became apparent that, when inoculated into germ-free rats, certain strains of oral streptococci were cariogenic whilst others were not. The most distinguishing characteristic of the cariogenic strains was their ability to form extracellular polysaccharides of the dextran type from sucrose. They also build up and store intracellular polysaccharides of the amylopectic type (Fitzgerald 1968).

Dental plaque can contain as much as 10 per cent of its dry weight as polysaccharide; part of this is intracellular, part extracellular, and both are produced by the micro-organisms of the plaque.

Intracellular Polysaccharide

Several species cultivated from plaque have been found to produce large amounts of intracellular polysaccharide of the amylopectin or glycogen type. Plaque from caries-active subjects shows a greater proportion of cultivatable micro-organisms capable of forming intracellular polysaccharide than plaque from caries-free subjects (Gibbons and Socransky 1962).

The intracellular store of polysaccharide can readily be degraded to organic acids when exogenous supplies of substrate are not available for energy purposes. Thus, intracellular polysaccharides could be formed by the plaque micro-organisms when suitable exogenous carbohydrate is abundant and used up during periods of scarcity, so prolonging the period when the plaque is at a low pH. This facet of plaque metabolism is of possible importance in the aetiology of dental caries and will be influenced by dietary factors.

Extracellular Polysaccharides

When strains of oral streptococci described as cariogenic—since they produce caries in germ-free animals—are grown in media containing sucrose, they produce large amounts of extracellular polysaccharides (Gibbons and Banghart 1967). Such polysaccharides are mainly polymers of glucose (dextrans) with smaller amounts of fructose polymers (levans). Analysis of dental plaque shows the presence of both dextrans and levans, but the levans are hydrolyzed and metabolized more readily than dextrans and therefore more dextran than levan accumulates in plaque. In vitro cariogenic streptococci produce more adherent polysaccharides than do 'non-cariogenic' streptococci when grown in the presence of sucrose. Also, most of the known cariogenic streptococci produce dextran from sucrose but not in any great quantity from other sugars. This suggests that in these organisms the dextran–sucrose enzyme system is involved, which demands the presence of sucrose as a substrate for the formation of 1- to 6-linked dextrans.

Therefore, polysaccharide synthesis in dental plaque may be an important factor in the production of dental caries. The accumulation of intracellular polysaccharide may provide a source of carbohydrate readily metabolizable to organic acids when an external source of substrate is not available. The synthesis of extracellular polysaccharide may be important for two reasons. First, levans found in the presence of sucrose are readily metabolized to acids, and second, dextrans are not readily broken down and hence will help to build up the bulk of the plaque since they readily form adherent deposits. Thus plaque formation depends to some extent on the production of extracellular dextran.

Protective Factors in Food

The idea that certain natural foods might contain protective factors against caries has been put forward from time to time. Osborn and Noriskin (1937) were probably the first to suggest this based upon their observations of low caries experience among the South African Bantus living in their native kraals compared with that of similar groups living in towns. The overall carbohydrate consumption of the two groups was similar but the native diet was mainly unrefined mealie meal whilst that of the town dwellers included white bread and sucrose. Other workers have repeated the in vitro methods of the Osborn team using more refined quantitative methods and have obtained overwhelming evidence that unrefined foods do contain substances which lower the solubility rate of teeth in vitro (Andlaw 1960; Jenkins et al. 1959). In brown flour these substances have been identified with the organically bound phosphates, mostly phytate (Grenby 1967; Jenkins et al. 1959) which appears to bind to the enamel surface. Data on the effect of brown bread on caries in man are extremely difficult to obtain since those who avoid white bread are frequently selective with respect to other aspects of their diet. Turner and Vickery (1966) compared the dental health of 103 British children who had received wholemeal bread for a minimum of five years with the published data for caries incidence in various control groups of fiuoridation studies. The figures showed clearly the lower incidence of caries in the wholemeal group. However, many variables were involved and there was an absence of information on sugar intake. Thus, although there are theoretical grounds for expecting brown bread to be less cariogenic than white bread, animal experiments have not supported this conclusion.

Antibacterial Factors in Unrefined Cereals

Several groups of workers have found that the inclusion of oat hulls as 25 per cent of a cariogenic diet reduces caries in experimental animals (Buttner and Muhler 1959). Madsen and Edmonds (1962) reported similar results with hulls from rice, peanuts, cotton seeds and pecan. The mechanical effects of these hulls were eliminated and the ash was inactive. Thus, Taketa and Phillips (1957) concluded that some organic constituent was responsible for reducing caries. They found that ethanol extracts of oat hulls contained substances which inhibited the growth of lactobacilli and reduced caries in rats. The oat hulls contained water-soluble substances which reduced enamel solubility, and it seems more likely that this action was responsible for the caries reduction than antibacterial factors (Jenkins 1968).

Protective Factors in Crude Sugars

In vitro experiments have shown that crude cane juice contains a complex mixture of substances which reduce the solubility rate of enamel (Jenkins et al. 1959). Black treacle (molasses) still contained much of the activity of the cane juice with the additional effect of a high concentration (0.5 per cent) of calcium derived from the lime added to the cane juice at one stage of the purification. On theoretical grounds, therefore, it might be expected that molasses would be less cariogenic than an equivalent amount of pure sucrose, but there is no clinical evidence for this. Strälfors (1966) reported that diets containing brown sugar produced less caries in hamsters than those with equivalent levels of pure sucrose, thus supporting the suggestion that brown sugar contains active protective factors. König and Muhlemann (1967) pointed out that crystals of crude sugar consisted of coarser particles than the pure sucrose. Further experiments by König and Muhlemann (1967) showed clearly that the particle size was the important factor since similar levels of caries incidence occurred when both sugars were ground to the same size.

Phosphates

Phosphates have been tested in experimental animals and in clinical trials on man as possible caries-preventive agents. When inorganic phosphates have been added to cariogenic diets of rats or hamsters, a significant cariostatic action has been demonstrated. The mechanism of action of phosphates in caries reduction is uncertain but the conclusion of numerous workers points to a local rather than a systemic effect. There is a significant difference in the cariostatic effect of phosphate ingested orally compared to that administered to rats by stomach tube (McClure 1965). The local effect may be related to four factors:

1. The ability of phosphate ions to reduce the rate of dissolution of hydroxyapatite.

2. The ability of supersaturated solutions of phosphate ions to reprecipitate calcium phosphate in partially demineralized enamel (Silverstone 1977).

3. The ability of phosphates to buffer organic acids formed by fermentation of plaque microflora.

4. The ability of the phosphate ion to desorb proteins from the enamel surface and thus modify the pellicle (Pruitt et al. 1940).

Although much experimental effort has been focused on the use of inorganic phosphates, both soluble and insoluble (König et al. 1967), the use of organic phosphates has attracted increasing attention. The use of phosphates as cariostatic agents is based on a number of hypotheses:

1. That it is possible to raise the concentration of this ion in plaque either directly or through saliva by increasing the intake of phosphate by mouth.

2. That some phosphates can be adsorbed onto the enamel surface (Jenkins et al. 1959).

3. That the ingestion of diets rich in phosphates will affect the chemical composition of teeth.

It was observed by Bowen (1969) that the drop in pH values in plaque could be prevented effectively by the inclusion of one per cent calcium glycerophosphate in a test sugar solution. Further work in monkeys on a diet containing one per cent calcium glycerophosphate showed a reduction in caries compared with controls and a reduction in the quantity of plaque (Brown 1972).

In recent years calcium sucrose phosphate has been tested as an additive to sucrose. It reduces the solubility of enamel in vitro as does phytate. A clinical trial was carried out in Australia (Harris et al. 1967) on 1,500 children aged 5 to 17 years. An overall reduction of 20 per cent in caries was claimed, with a 35 per cent reduction on proximal surfaces of posterior teeth. This study has been criticized because the sucrose phosphate contained significant amounts of fluoride.

143

Trace Elements

The role of water-borne fluorides is the only factor fully established to reduce caries significantly. This has been discussed in Chapter 4. The evidence that other trace elements influence caries is far less convincing. However, limited epidemiological evidence has suggested that molybdenum and vanadium may reduce caries and selenium increase it. Hadjimarkos (1966) has pointed out that fluoride is the only trace element which is largely obtained from water and that food sources should be considered before concluding that a trace element is related to caries. This has been done for molybdenum and selenium but not for vanadium. Molybdenum is present in vegetables and its concentration can be increased by growing them on alkaline soil. This factor offers a possible means of increasing molybdenum intake.

Vitamin B$_6$

The only vitamin which has been considered recently in relation to caries is vitamin B$_6$ which, in large doses (10 to 20 times the normal daily intake), has been reported to reduce caries both in animals and human subjects (Hillman et al. 1962) although this is not well established. However, this is more correctly considered as a pharmacological use of a vitamin, presumably exerted by toxic effects on oral bacteria.

Fats and Caries

Several workers have shown that increasing the proportion of fat in the diet reduces the cariogenic effect of sugar. The mechanism is not certain but may possibly be physical. A layer of fat surrounding carbohydrate food or covering the plaque prevents access of substrate to bacteria, or of acid to enamel. Milk has sometimes been considered to be cariogenic. In vitro experiments and studies on the effect of milk on plaque pH have given little support to the idea that it has any local effect in favouring caries (Jenkins and Ferguson 1966). In fact, there were indications that milk would reduce the effect of sugar. The protein, calcium and phosphate acted as protective factors and the lactose of milk supported only feeble acid production in plaque in vivo.

Cocoa and Chocolate

There is evidence that cocoa and chocolate contain protective factors. It is not suggested that the overall effect of chocolate would be to reduce caries but merely that the sugar in chocolate might be less damaging than similar amounts of sugar in other forms. Animal experiments by Strälfors (1966) showed that as little as two per cent cocoa in the diet reduced caries in hamsters by more than 40 per cent. He showed that the fat of cocoa did not reduce caries but, contrary to work with other fats, increased it. Fractionation of cocoa extracts and tests on various known constituents showed that several of them were active in reducing hamster caries.

Apart from foods containing fluorides, it cannot be said that any group has been shown to have a definite protective effect against caries in man. Nevertheless the evidence presented suggests that more work is justified on several substances such as organic and inorganic phosphates, molybdenum and vanadium. In addition, several foods deserve more investigation.

Replacement of Sucrose by Other Sweeteners

Trials of sucrose substitutes have been carried out, largely in Scandinavia and Switzerland.

Sorbitol

Sorbitol is the sweetener used in many diabetic preparations. Although only about half as sweet as sucrose, and less sweet than the inexpensive glucose, it has advantages as a non-cariogenic sweetener. A mouth rinse with a 50 per cent solution of sorbitol or chewing candies made with sorbitol produced little or no drop in pH (Frostell 1964). Sorbitol is fermented by practically all strains of *Streptococcus mutans* to give a final pH of below 5.0. Numerous studies have shown that when sorbitol is applied to dental plaque in situ or in vitro very little alteration in the pH of the plaque occurs,

145

unlike the situation with most sugars which cause a dramatic and rapid drop in the pH of plaque. Presumably the reason that sorbitol does not lower appreciably the pH in plaque is because the rate of fermentation of sorbitol by *S. mutans* is much slower than that of other fermentable mono- and disaccharides. This permits salivary buffers to neutralize acid end-products as they are formed. Sorbitol or partially hydrolyzed hydrogenated starches (containing about 28 per cent sorbitol) have been tested for their cariogenicity by several independent investigators. Sorbitol has been compared with sucrose and other carbohydrates and was found to cause much less caries and a reduction in plaque accumulation relative to sucrose. Sorbitol is absorbed more slowly than glucose and causes diarrhoea in some individuals, presumably by the osmotic effect of unabsorbed sorbitol retaining water in the intestine.

Xylitol

Xylitol has a similar degree of sweetness to sucrose and occurs naturally in a number of foods such as bananas and mushrooms. The only factor which appears to limit the dosage of xylitol is the phenomenon of osmotic diarrhoea, or soft faeces. As with sorbitol, individual susceptibility to this inconvenience varies and tolerance of xylitol is markedly increased by frequent dosage. During long-term trials, Scheinin et al. (1974) found a notable absence of diarrhoea and other side-effects. Only one of 52 participants in the xylitol group withdrew from the study, and this was because of diarrhoea. Xylitol does not lower plaque pH appreciably and is of very low cariogenicity when fed to rats. When xylitol was incorporated into human diets, the plaque weight was reduced significantly compared with sucrose diets. Xylitol in human diets has proved to be less cariogenic than sucrose or fructose (Scheinin et al. 1974).

Aspartame

Aspartame (aspartyl phenylalanine methyl ester) is about 160 times sweeter than sucrose in aqueous solution. It has been suggested that this dipeptide has potential as a low caloric sweetener. Poor stability in acidic solution may limit its use in carbonated beverages and fruit products. This instability manifests itself as a loss of sweetness during storage and possibly during hot processing. No long-range toxicity results are yet available for this compound. Some safety studies have been completed and to date no undesirable results have been observed according to its manufacturers.

Saccharin

Of the sugar substitutes, saccharin has been known for the longest time and is undoubtedly the most widely used. Saccharin is between 200 and 700 times as sweet as sucrose and is heat-stable. It is excreted in the urine almost without metabolic alteration. The Food and Drug Administration in the USA has set limits on the use of saccharin, being 1 g per day for a 155 lb person, citing evidence that rodents develop bladder tumours when fed extremely high levels. Saccharin has been removed from the list of food additives generally recognized as safe.

Cyclamates

Sodium cyclamate is approximately 30 times as sweet as sucrose, has a pleasantly sweet taste and is freely soluble in water. Tests have shown that cyclamates are metabolized and excreted in an unchanged form in man. Cyclamates have been shown to induce chromosome breaks in both leucocytes and monolayer cultures of human skin and cancer cells in in vitro studies on human cells. Since August 1970, sale of cyclamates has been banned in the USA. Cyclamates used in dosages 50 times the daily maximum recommended for humans were found to induce bladder cancer in rats. Little evidence, however, implicates the role of cyclamates in human disease since, prior to 1970, cyclamates were without any influence on bladder carcinoma rates in the USA.

Monellin

Monellin is a soluble protein isolated from serendipity berries which are obtained from a tropical plant (*Dioscoreophyllum cumminsii* Diels). Monellin is about 3,000 times sweeter than sucrose, the sweet sensation persisting in the mouth for an unusual length of time. A limitation to its possible industrial use is the fact that on standing at room temperature the purified protein loses its sweetness within 24 hours.

In order for a sugar substitute to be an acceptable sweetener with commercial potential, it must satisfy four important criteria:

1. It must have sufficient sweetening power.

2. The product must be non-toxic.

3. In order to be commercially viable the product must be reasonably inexpensive.

4. The substance must be thermostable so as to remain unchanged over the range of cooking temperatures.

Many of the sugar substitutes have no practical use as sweetening agents because they do not satisfy all the above criteria. The imposed limitation in the amount of saccharin for consumption in the USA and the withdrawal of cyclamates highlights the problem in this field.

Conclusion

During the past four decades there has been an increasing awareness of the effects of diet on dental health. However, further information is required to understand fully the nutritional requirements of the tooth and supporting structures. With respect to dietary control of dental caries, the major problem is not what to do to prevent caries but how to persuade the patient to comply with sound dietary advice. There is a real need to study dental caries not only as a pathological entity but also as a social problem. Social scientists must be encouraged to study the attitudes of people to dental health and the behavioural factors involved.

References

Andlaw, R. J., *J. Dent. Res.*, 1960, **39**, 1200.
Bowen, W. H., *Br. Dent. J.*, 1969, **126**, 506.

Bowen, W. H., *Caries Res.*, 1972, **6**, 43.

Bradford, E. W. and Crabb, H. S. M., *Br. Dent. J.*, 1961, **111**, 273.

Buttner, W. and Muhler, J. C., *J. Dent. Res.*, 1959, **38**, 823.

Fitzgerald, R. J., *Alabam. J. Med. Sci.*, 1968, **5**, 239.

Frostell, G., in *Nutrition and Caries Prevention, Symposium of the Swedish Nutrition Foundation III*, X. Blix (Ed.), pp 60–66, Almquist and Wiksell, Stockholm, 1964.

Frostell, G., Keyes, P. and Larson, R. H., *J. Nutr.*, 1967, **93**, 65.

Gibbons, R. J. and Socransky, S. S., *Arch. Oral Biol.*, 1962, **7**, 73.

Green, R. M. and Hartlęs, R. L., *Br. J. Nutr.*, 1967, **21**, 225.

Green, R. M. and Hartles, R. L., *Caries Res.*, 1969, **3**, 208.

Grenby, T. H., *Arch. Oral Biol.*, 1963, **8**, 27.

Grenby, T. H., *Arch. Oral Biol.*, 1967, **12**, 513.

Guggenheim, B., König, K. G., Herzog, E. and Muhlemann, H. R., *Helv. Odont. Acta*, 1966, **10**, 101.

Gustafsson, B. E., Quensel, C. E., Lanke, L. S., Ludquist, C., Grahnen, H., Bonow, B. E. and Krasse, B., *Acta Odont. Scand.*, 1954, **11**, 232.

Hadjimarkos, D. M., *Nature*, 1966, **201**, 1137.

Harris, R., *J. Dent. Res.*, 1963, **42**, 1387.

Harris, R., Schamschula, R. G., Gregory, G., Roots, M. and Beveridge, J., *Aust. Dent. J.*, 1967, **12**, 105.

Hillman, R. W., Cabaud, P. G. and Scherone, R. A., *Am. J. Clin. Nutr.*, 1962, **10**, 512.

Jenkins, G. N., *Alabam. J. Med. Sci.*, 1968, **5**, 276.

Jenkins, G. N. and Ferguson, D. B., *Br. Dent. J.*, 1966, **120**, 472.

Jenkins, G. N., Forster, M. G., Speirs, R. L. and Kleinberg, I., *Br. Dent. J.*, 1959, **106**, 195.

König, K. G. and Muhlemann, H. R., *Arch. Oral Biol.*, 1967, **12**, 1297.

Ludwig. T. G., Denby, G. C. and Struthers, W. G., *N.Z. Dent. J.*, 1960, **56**, 174.

Madsen, K. O. and Edmonds, E. J., *J. Dent. Res.*, 1962, **41**, 404.

Mansbridge, J. N., *Br. Dent. J.*, 1960, **109**, 343.

Marthaler, T. M. and Froesch, E. R., *Br. Dent. J.*, 1967, **123**, 597.

McClure, F. J., *Arch. Oral Biol.*, 1965, **10**, 1011.

Mellanby, H. and Mellanby, M., *Br. Med. J.*, 1950, **1**, 1341.

Osborn, T. W. B. and Noriskin, J. N., *J. Dent. Res.*, 1937, **16**, 431.

Pruitt, K. M., Jamieson, A. D. and Caldwell, R. C., *Nature*, 1970, **225**, 1249.

Scheinin, A., Makinen, K. K. and Ylitalo, K., *Acta Odont. Scand.*, 1974, **32**, 383.

Silverstone, L. M., *Caries Res.*, 1977, **11** (Suppl. 1), 59.

Stephan, R. M., *J. Dent. Res.*, 1966, **45**, 1551.

Strälfors, A., *Arch. Oral Biol.*, 1966, **12**, 959.

Sullivan, H. R. and Harris, R., *Aust. Dent. J.*, 1958, **3**, 311.

Preventive Dentistry

Taketa, F. and Phillips, P. H., *J. Am. Diet. Assoc.*, 1957, **33**, 575.
Takeuchi, M., *Int. Dent. J.,* 1961, **11, 443.**
Toverud, G., *J. Am. Diet. Assoc.*, 1950, **26**, 673.
Turner, E. and Vickery, K. O. A., *Z. Vit. Zivil.*, 1966, **53**, 3.

9. The Caries Preventive Regimen—A Summary

In this book I have attempted to cover a number of aspects of caries prevention that can be adopted in general dental practice. To practise competent caries prevention it is necessary first to have some relevant basic knowledge of the disease mechanisms and the tissues they affect. Only by understanding the essential points in the initiation and progress of the disease one is attempting to prevent can the best be derived from preventive techniques.

Fluoride Supplementation

The ingestion of an optimum level of fluoride during tooth development forms the basis for any successful caries preventive regimen. Where the domestic water supply contains an optimum fluoride concentration of 1.0 ppm, either naturally or by artificial means, the population will receive adequate fluoride. The reduction in dental caries is greater than 50 per cent in permanent teeth (Backer-Dirks 1974) and slightly less for primary teeth (Scherp 1971). This is a true public health measure, since no individual effort is required on behalf of the population. The percentage of domestic water supplies containing adequate levels of fluoride varies greatly from country to country. For example, in the USA, of the 213 million population in 1975, about 177 million persons received public water supplies. Of these, approximately 59 per cent received water supplies that are fluoridated either naturally or artificially. In the UK, however, only about six per cent of the population receive fluoridated water.

Therefore, for those persons who do not consume fluoridated drinking water during the period of tooth formation, fluoride supplements must be recommended as an essential basis for a caries preventive regimen.

Fluoride Tablets

Ideally a fluoride tablet should be sucked in order to increase the topical fluoride effect. Tablets that contain 0.25 mg fluoride ion should be available to comply with the new recommendations for fluoride supplementation given in Chapter 2.

Fluoride Dosage

Pregnant Mothers

The evidence now available does not give support to the use of fluoride as a prenatal supplement for caries prevention.

From Birth to Six Months of Age

It is recommended that no fluoride supplementation be given during this period.

Six Months to Eighteen Months of Age

Where the local water supply is deficient with respect to fluoride, having less than 0.2 ppm, a daily tablet containing 0.25 mg fluoride ion is recommended. If the local water supply has more than 0.2 ppm fluoride, no additional fluoride should be given.

Eighteen Months to Three Years of Age

Where the local drinking water is fluoride deficient, a daily supplementation of 0.5 mg fluoride ion should be given. If the local water supply contains 0.2 to 0.4 ppm fluoride, the daily fluoride tablet should contain only 0.25 mg fluoride ion. If the local water supply contains more than 0.5 ppm fluoride, no additional fluoride should be given.

From Three to Six Years of Age

Where the local water supply has less than 0.2 ppm fluoride, a daily fluoride supplementation of 0.75 mg fluoride ion should be given. If the local water contains 0.2 to 0.4 ppm fluoride, the daily dosage should be reduced to 0.5 mg fluoride ion. No fluoride tablets should be given if the local water supply contains 0.5 ppm fluoride or more.

From Six Years of Age

The full daily supplementation of 1 mg fluoride ion should be given if the fluoride concentration of the local water is less than 0.2 ppm. Where the water supply contains 0.2 to 0.4 ppm fluoride, the daily dosage should be reduced to 0.75 mg fluoride ion. This should be reduced further to 0.5 mg fluoride ion daily if the local water supply contains 0.4 to 0.6 ppm fluoride. With a fluoride concentration of 0.6 to 0.8 ppm, the daily dosage should be 0.25 mg fluoride ion. No supplementation should be given if the local water supply contains more than 0.8 ppm fluoride.

Plaque Control

Dental plaque is the major aetiological factor in caries and periodontal disease. Chewing fibrous foods between meals does not prevent plaque formation. In addition, plaque still forms on tooth surfaces of monkeys even when fed their entire diet by stomach tube (Bowen 1969). The efficient removal of plaque from tooth surfaces forms a very important part of preventive dentistry.

Toothbrushing

The toothbrush is the major instrument for plaque removal. A disclosing technique is essential since there is little hope of removing a film which is invisible at the start of the operation.

Frequency. It is far better to clean the teeth once a day thoroughly than quickly and inefficiently after every meal. If a once daily regimen is followed, the brushing period should be in the evening just before retiring to bed

The toothbrush. Toothbrushes should be replaced frequently.

153

Preventive Dentistry

The average life of a toothbrush is approximately three months. The most popular type of brush has a straight, semirigid handle with a small head about one inch long. The bristles are about half an inch long and the tufts of bristles are trimmed to uniform height. Most bristles are made of nylon. Patients with delicate or diseased gingival tissues should use a soft toothbrush with 250 μm diameter filaments. The kind of toothbrush a patient uses depends on his preference. Studies on brush design have not revealed any superior type.

Use of the toothbrush by children. Children under seven years of age are not always able to master an effective toothbrushing technique, so it is essential to have a parent carry out the major part of the brushing. Although seven different methods of brushing were evaluated at the World Workshop in Periodontics (Ramfjord et al. 1966), the participants could not recommend any one method as being better than others.

Mechanical toothbrushes. The effectiveness of electric toothbrushes is similar to those used manually but their use is especially indicated for the handicapped patient. Battery-operated models become less effective with power loss due to infrequent changing of batteries.

Dental Floss

Plaque will remain between the teeth in spite of careful and efficient use of a toothbrush. Therefore, the patient must be made aware of the relevance of dental floss as the only decisive way of removing plaque from interproximal regions.

Rather than introduce flossing techniques immediately, it is often wise to instruct a patient in the correct use of a toothbrush and introduce him to disclosing techniques. The patient is then told to practise plaque control and report on the effectiveness at the next visit. Usually, at the next appointment, the patient will complain that he is failing to remove stained plaque from interproximal sites. Thus, the patient has identified the problem for himself. This is then the stage at which to introduce flossing techniques, since motivation will be high.

The Caries Preventive Regimen—A Summary

Topical Fluorides

Topical fluoride therapy can be broadly divided into two main regimens, 'low potency–high frequency' and 'high potency–low frequency'. The frequent exposure of teeth to low levels of fluoride is in direct contrast to the annual or biannual application of topical preparations containing 1.2 to 2.5 per cent fluorides. Frequent fluoride ingestion is necessary to sustain a circulating fluoride level in the blood and provide bioavailable fluoride for incorporation into developing tooth structure (Parkins 1977). Oral micro-organisms are directly affected by fluoride concentrations from high frequency preparations. Plaque also accumulates fluoride in amounts which are potentially high enough to have an effect on the adjacent enamel surface and the plaque micro-organisms. For fluoride to inhibit acid production by micro-organisms and to become bound into plaque deposits it must be repeatedly present in the oral cavity (Parkins 1977).

High Potency–Low Frequency

All available evidence suggests that an acidulated phosphate fluoride (APF) gel should be used on a biannual basis. The frequency of use depends on the recall system used in the dental office. For a six-month recall system, biannual applications are advisable. If children are seen on a four-month recall plan, topical fluorides can be employed three times a year. Selection of the correct tray type is important as was stressed in Chapter 5. Air-cushion trays (Ion Brand, 3M Company, Minnesota) are excellent with respect to both fluoride uptake by tooth enamel and patient acceptance. The only disadvantage is that each arch must be treated separately. Centrays (Pacemaker Corp, Portland, Oregon) preformed disposable trays are well accepted by young patients. Both arches can be treated at one time, and good fluoride uptake results from their use. Recently new Centrays have been introduced which are specifically lower moulds and blue in colour. Therefore, a pair of trays will consist of a white upper tray and a blue lower tray. These are highly recommended by the author.

155

High Frequency–Low Potency

A variety of fluoride-containing mouth rinses are available for administration on a daily to weekly basis. The use of fluoride mouth rinses has been shown to produce significant reductions in caries incidence (see Chapter 6) and may be an answer to the problems caused by insufficient professional manpower and excessive costs that currently hinder topical fluoride programmes.

Unsupervised use of a fluoridated dentifrice in low fluoride areas produces a small but significant reduction in caries incidence—a reduction in DMFS of approximately 20 per cent. Because this technique does not depend upon professional or supervised care, it represents a very useful and important part of a caries preventive regimen. Most fluoride-containing dentifrices contain 1,000 ppm fluoride. Significant caries reductions have also been observed with the combined use of a fluoride-containing dentifrice and a topical fluoride programme (Muhler et al. 1967; Scola and Ostrom 1969).

Home Fluoride Treatment

For children or adults with problems of severe or rampant caries, an intensive course of fluoride applications may be prescribed for home use. The daily home use of a fluoride gel containing 0.6 per cent fluoride ion has been recommended (Wei 1976). A number of APF gels are now commercially available for home use (Pacemaker Corp., Lorvic Corp., and Hoyt Corp.). The use of suitable trays is recommended in the application of fluoride gels as part of the home fluoride treatment. A prescription for 250 ml of 0.6 per cent fluoride ion APF gel should last approximately three months. Home fluoride treatment should be commenced prior to, and continued during, restorative treatment. Once control of the active phase has been achieved, therapy should be continued with lower potency fluoride supplements such as fluoride mouthrinses. Home fluoride treatment is contraindicated in young children who may swallow a significant portion of the fluoride agent. This could lead to the possibility of enamel fluorosis.

The Caries Preventive Regimen—A Summary

Dietary Counselling

Specific time must be set aside for a session devoted to dietary counselling. Ideally, this should take place in a patient education room and not in the dental office. This education room should be equipped with appropriate food visual aids and furnished in a pleasant and comfortable manner. These factors will help the patient realize that nutritional counselling is a specialized dental service and requires a specific appointment as does, for example, a restorative session.

There are two visits which require a significant amount of time (Nizel 1972): the original counselling visit and the recall visit for re-evaluation. Prior to the first visit, a detailed medical and dental history is obtained together with relevant details of the patient's social background and dietary habits. This is essential in order to appreciate the attitudes, motivations and environmental factors which influence the patient's food selection and eating habits.

A detailed diet-sheet should then be obtained after the patient has been shown the correct method for recording relevant details. The value of the diet-sheet is not in its accuracy, which is usually poor (Holloway 1963), but in providing a discussion topic for dentist, dietician and parent/patient. The sheet should contain details of all that the patient has eaten or drunk over a three-day period. The three-day period should include a weekend since parents will have more control over the eating habits of their child than during schooldays and a more accurate diet record will be obtained. Another important point to stress tactfully is truthful recording. Two aspects of the diet-sheet are important: first, the type of food or drink and the form in which it is taken, and second, the time at which it is consumed.

When the completed diet record is returned at the next appointment, it should be carefully checked. Although there are a number of ways to make use of diet records, a simple, qualitative, analytical approach is probably the most satisfactory. The aim is to restrict the number of intakes of refined carbohydrates. It is almost impossible to avoid this during the main meals, but the important factor is to reduce and modify eating habits between meals.

Eating between Meals

Considerable evidence demonstrates that sucrose-containing foods taken as snacks between meals are highly cariogenic. Children should be encouraged to eat a well-balanced meal at the correct time so as to eliminate the necessity for snacks. Since between-meal eating by many children cannot be eliminated, snacks low in sucrose content should be offered, e.g. fresh fruit, vegetables, crackers, cheese, and nuts.

It may also be unrealistic to recommend the total elimination of sweets for all children. A compromise is to select a specific time once a week when the child can consume all the sweets he wishes.

Diet Evaluation

The parent, and child if old enough, must be made aware of the cariogenic aspects of the diet as displayed in the diet record. A general statement to the effect that sweet foods must be eliminated will be of no effect whatsoever. The dentist should draw the patient's attention to the cariogenic aspects of the diet by, for example, placing a heavy red circle around the relevant foodstuffs. It should then be explained that each red circle represents an 'acid attack' on the teeth. At this stage, the dentist should re-enforce the fundamental details of caries formation so that the patient is aware of the significance of the 'acid attack'.

In this way, a parent might see that her son has nine 'acid attacks' a day. This will present a specific target for the parent and in future diet record sheets they can see if their efforts are rewarded by a reduction in the number of acid attacks shown on the record sheet. This is a more positive approach than a general statement aimed at a reduction in fermentable carbohydrate intake. It does not really matter what type of scoring system is used provided that it can initially convey information to the patient and parent and later give feedback on whether their approach to the problem has been positive. To see the number of acid attacks reduced from nine to three over a single day is an achievement on behalf of the patient and parent and can be a significant motivation factor.

The Caries Preventive Regimen—A Summary

A personalized evaluation sheet is prepared by the dentist. The evaluation sheet should discuss the patient's diet from the standpoint of general nutrition as well as from the dental outlook. The number of acid attacks occurring on each day of the diet record should be mentioned as well as the significance of acid in dental disease. Positive recommendations should be made, e.g. substitution of cariogenic snack foods by more suitable foodstuffs. The dentist should be able to arrive at a well-balanced diet that will be both practical and acceptable to the patient. A copy of the evaluation sheet should be given to the parent and a copy retained in the patient's notes together with the diet record sheets. Ideally, this procedure should be repeated after six weeks to see whether there has been a change in the patient's dietary habits.

Fissure Sealants

Chapter 7 was devoted to the development, rationale and use of pit and fissure sealants. Fissure caries occurs earlier than caries on smooth surfaces, and the occlusal surface is least benefited by fluoride. Most epidemiological studies report that occlusal caries accounts for 50 per cent or more of the total caries experience up to 18 years of age. Jackson (1974) stated that fissure caries contributes approximately 80 per cent of total attacks by 15 years of age. Jackson (1973) has calculated that if fissure sealants achieved only 50 per cent prevention in a fluoride community, the need for restorations in permanent teeth by 15 years of age could be reduced by 74 per cent.

A Suggested Caries Preventive Regimen

Systemic Fluoride

If the patient resides in a non-fluoridated water area, the local water supply should be analysed to determine the natural fluoride content. If the fluoride content is less than 0.2 ppm, children should be advised to commence a fluoride supplementation regimen using sodium fluoride tablets. The dosage should comply with

159

the recommendations given in Chapter 2, Table 1. If the fluoride content of the local water supply is higher than 0.2 ppm, the dosage should be modified according to the recommendations. An adequate intake of systemic fluoride is an essential baseline to a caries preventive regimen. The fluoride tablet should ideally take a long time to dissolve in the mouth so as to benefit *from the topical fluoride effect.*

Toothbrushing

Toothbrushing should commence as soon as teeth begin to appear in the oral cavity. In fact, the gentle use of a small toothbrush on the gum pads prior to eruption of the first deciduous teeth often brings relief of symptoms associated with eruption. The use of toothpaste is optional at this stage. A fluoride-containing dentifrice should not be used until the child is four years of age, because children below this age are unable to expectorate satisfactorily. A parent should assist in toothbrushing until the child is capable of carrying this out himself, usually at about seven years of age. Efficient and thorough toothbrushing at all ages should be carried out at least once a day, ideally just prior to retiring for the night. Dental floss is an important adjunct but not necessarily so in the deciduous dentition since these teeth are often well spaced, and a young child is not likely to tolerate the rigour of flossing even if a parent is willing to carry out the technique. Flossing should be introduced during the mixed dentition stage and used initially with a disclosing technique. Patients of all ages should check the efficacy of their plaque control regimen by using disclosing techniques at regular intervals.

Dietary Counselling

A detailed diet-sheet should be obtained and scoring system employed to point out the number of 'acid attacks' that occur on each day of the diet recording. This gives the patient a specific goal and he can see whether his efforts have been rewarded by a reduction in this number at a later date.

The Caries Preventive Regimen—A Summary

Increasing the Resistance of the Teeth

Fissure Sealants

Ideally, occlusal surfaces should be fissure-sealed immediately after eruption into the mouth. The necessity for an increased etching time of two minutes with deciduous molars has been discussed in Chapter 7. The type of sealant employed is less important than the care and attention given to the etching phase. Salivary contamination of etched surfaces prior to application and polymerization of the resin must be avoided, and the air/water line to the triple spray must be free from contamination by oil and water vapour if a satisfactory bond is to occur Although all occlusal surfaces should ideally be sealed, the first permanent molars must certainly be protected since they have a high susceptibility to occlusal caries. Sealants should be checked at recall examinations and, if a deficiency is suspected, a further supply of resin can be added after re-etching the occlusal surface. The re-etching regimen will show to what extent the surface is covered by sealant. It is difficult to detect clinically the presence of sealants after they have been in situ for a year or more. A new Enamel Bond sealant (3M Dental Products) has recently been introduced, with titanium dioxide incorporated in the resin to give a brilliant white colour to the sealant, which aids in its identification. Similarly, Alpha Seal (Amalgamated Dental Co.) has a UV light fluorescent agent which can be detected on occlusal surfaces when examined by means of the Alpha-Lite (Amalgamated Dental Co.) UV light beam.

Topical Fluorides: High Potency–Low Frequency

Prophylaxis. Use a fluoride-containing prophylaxis paste (APF) with a rubber cup for initial cleaning of enamel surfaces.

Gels. Use an acidulated phosphate fluoride (APF) gel for topical application allowing the fluoride to remain in contact with the teeth for four minutes. After the exposure time, excess gel should be wiped off the teeth using gauze and the patient should not rinse his mouth, eat or drink for 30 minutes.

Thixotropic materials. Evidence is accumulating to indicate that the new thixotropic APF gels may have advantages with respect to penetration of interproximal contact sites (Silverstone 1977). Thus, the new thixotropic fluoride gels should be employed in the topical fluoride regimen (e.g. Gel II by Pacemaker).

Flavours. Taste is an important consideration and some of the newer flavours of APF gels are acceptable to children (e.g. chocolate flavour Gel II by Pacemaker Corp., Portland, Oregon).

Trays. An efficient tray system for application of fluoride gels must be employed. Air-cushion trays (Ion Brand, 3M Dental Products) are extremely comfortable for children, produce good contact with enamel surfaces, and can be connected to the high speed aspirator by plastic tubing for efficient moisture control. However, only one dental arch can be treated at one time because of their size and, therefore, two separate four-minute exposures must be carried out in order to treat a whole mouth. Centrays (Pacemaker Corp) are excellent disposable trays, well accepted by patients, and fit the dental arch well, especially since the recent introduction of separate upper and lower moulds, each colour-coded.

The topical fluoride regimen should be repeated at each recall visit. If any restorative treatment is required, this should be performed first, and the topical application carried out as the last item on the treatment plan. In this way, any new enamel–amalgam or enamel–composite interfaces can be exposed to the fluoride gel where some beneficial ion exchange can take place.

Topical Fluorides: Low Potency–High Frequency

Dentifrices. After four years of age, patients should automatically be advised in the use of a fluoride-containing dentifrice. Although the reduction in caries incidence is small, it is nevertheless significant, especially since no professional time is involved. Non-staining monofluorophosphate is preferred to stannous fluoride pastes which stain.

Fluoride mouth rinses. If a patient has a specific caries problem, or if he is undergoing orthodontic therapy, especially with fixed appliances, a fluoride mouth-rinsing regimen is recommended. Although both daily and weekly regimens have produced good results in clinical trials, a weekly regimen with a 0.2 per cent sodium fluoride solution is preferable since it requires less patient co-operation than a daily routine. A specific time period for the regimen should be prescribed and the situation assessed at the end of this time.

References

Backer-Dirks, O., *Caries Res.*, 1974, **8** (Suppl.), 2.

Bowen, W. H., *Br. Dent. J.*, 1969, **126**, 159.

Holloway, P. J., *Nutrition*, 1963, **17**, 1.

Jackson, D., *Br. Dent. J.*, 1973, **134**, 480.

Jackson, D., *Br. Dent. J.*, 1974, **137**, 91.

Muhler, J. C., Spear, L. B., Bixler, D. and Stookey, G. K., *J. Am. Dent. Assoc.*, 1967, **75**, 1402.

Nizel, A. E., *Nutrition in Preventive Dentistry: Science and Practice*, W. B. Saunders, Philadelphia, 1972.

Parkins, F. M., *J. Prev. Dent.*, 1977, 4, 30.

Ramfjord, S. P., Kerr, D. A. and Ash, M. A. (Eds), *World Workshop in Periodontics*, University of Michigan, Ann Arbor, 1966.

Scherp, H. W., *Science*, 1971, **173**, 1199.

Scola, F. P. and Ostrom, C. A., *J. Am. Dent. Assoc.*, 1969, **78**, 594.

Silverstone, L. M., *Proc. Six. Cong. Int. Assoc. Dent. Child.*, San Francisco, California, 1977.

Wei, S. H. Y., *Fluorides: An Update for Dental Practice*, S. Moss and S. H. Y. Wei (Eds), Medcom, New York, 1976.